PHARMACOLOGY - RESEARCH, SAFETY TESTING AND REGULATION

DRUG COMPOUNDING

BACKGROUND, ISSUES AND FDA OVERSIGHT

PHARMACOLOGY - RESEARCH, SAFETY TESTING AND REGULATION

Additional books in this series can be found on Nova's website under the Series tab.

Additional E-books in this series can be found on Nova's website under the E-book tab.

PHARMACOLOGY - RESEARCH, SAFETY TESTING AND REGULATION

DRUG COMPOUNDING

BACKGROUND, ISSUES AND FDA OVERSIGHT

MARTTI BRAM
EDITOR

nova publishers
New York

For permission to use material from this book please contact us:
Telephone 631-231-7269; Fax 631-231-8175
Web Site: http://www.novapublishers.com

Library of Congress Cataloging-in-Publication Data

ISBN: 978-1-63117-360-8

Published by Nova Science Publishers, Inc. †New York

CONTENTS

PREFACE

Compounding has been traditionally defined as a process where a pharmacist or a physician combines, mixes, or alters ingredients to create a medication tailored to the needs of an individual patient. Traditionally compounded drugs (CDs) are made in response to an individual prescription from a licensed health provider in the context of a pharmacist's and health care professional's relationship with a specific patient. This book provides background information on CDs and non-traditional compounding pharmacies relevant to policy discussions. This book will also examine the FDA's regulation of drug compounding and will discuss relevant legal authorities. Specifically, the status of FDA's authority to oversee drug compounding, and the gaps, if any, between state and federal authority will be discussed, as well as how FDA has used its data and authority to oversee drug compounding, and the actions taken or planned by states or national pharmacy organizations to improve oversight of drug compounding.

Chapter 1 – Compounding has been traditionally defined as a process where a pharmacist or a physician combines, mixes, or alters ingredients to create a medication tailored to the needs of an individual patient. Traditionally compounded drugs (CDs) are made in response to an individual prescription from a licensed health provider in the context of a pharmacist's and health care professional's relationship with a specific patient. Some have suggested that certain activities not traditionally associated with compounding be considered compounding. Such activities include the large-scale production of drugs to ease certain drug shortages, to meet outsourcing needs of hospitals, and to supply physician-administered drugs. Non-traditional compounding may include (1) the production and shipping of large volume of drugs across state lines; (2) production of drugs that are copies of FDA-approved commercially available drugs; (3) provision of CD without a prescription for an individual patient to receive a compounded version and outside of a professional relationship; and (4) production of products to third parties, such as hospitals, clinics, physician offices, and home health providers. These activities could be considered more akin to manufacturing than traditional compounding, which is considered part of the traditional practice of pharmacy. Adverse events involving contaminated compounded drugs have drawn attention to the growing use of non-traditionally compounded drugs in health care delivery. Shortages of sterile generic drugs and hospital outsourcing are cited as causes of increased numbers of CDs produced by nontraditional compounders. Efforts to assess the risks and benefits of CDs on public health and safety are complicated by the lack of publicly available information, including the absence of a federal adverse event reporting requirement, and the lack of information about the number of drugs compounded, the types of drugs compounded, and the number of businesses in this market. Policymakers have raised questions regarding how best to improve the safety of CDs while maintaining patient access to needed medications. Drug compounding has historically been the focus of state governments through their regulation of pharmacies. Recently questions have arisen regarding the extent to which the federal government can regulate the practice of compounding through the Federal Food, Drug, and Cosmetic Act (FFDCA). Policy discussions include proposals to clarify federal oversight of high-risk activities and products, to improve federal and state coordination, and to increase use of existing federal authorities. This report provides background information on CDs and non-traditional compounding pharmacies relevant to policy discussions. This includes an overview of the 2012 fungal meningitis outbreak, recent safety alerts and recalls of compounded drugs, definitions of traditional compounding and non-traditional compounding, information on the CDs produced and by whom, information on the demand for non-traditional compounding, including the role of shortages of sterile injectable drugs, hospital out-sourcing, and patient and provider demand, and information on adverse events involving compounded drugs.

Chapter 2 – In light of the 2012 fungal meningitis outbreak, believed to have been caused by a contaminated compounded steroid injection, the regulation of human drug compounding has received significant attention. Drug compounding in its traditional form is the process of combining, mixing, or altering ingredients in order to create a medication for a particular patient. However, as illustrated by the entity that created the steroid medication linked with the meningitis outbreak, concerns have been raised about compounding pharmacies producing drugs on a larger scale. While drug compounding has historically been the focus of state governments through their regulation of pharmacies, questions have arisen regarding the extent the federal government can regulate the practice of compounding through the Food, Drug, and Cosmetic Act (FDCA). Federal authority over compounding largely stems from the FDCA, enacted in 1938, and its subsequent amendments, including the Food and Drug Administration Modernization Act (FDAMA) of 1997, which added compounding specific provisions to the FDCA in Section 503A. A First Amendment challenge to Section 503A's advertising provisions and a resulting Supreme Court decision has created a split amongst the federal courts regarding whether Section 503A has any legal effect. The legal uncertainty regarding Section 503A, coupled with Section 503A's basis in the FDCA's "new drug," "adulteration," and "misbranding" provisions lends to an examination of the scope of federal authority under the base statute. Courts appear to agree that the federal government can regulate compounding activity that is akin to manufacturing, and courts have afforded deference to the FDA's interpretation of when a compounder is acting like a manufacturer. However, uncertainty remains regarding the possible limits to the FDA's power to regulate traditional compounding activities. This report will examine the FDA's regulation of drug compounding and will discuss relevant legal authorities. The report will conclude by discussing potential limits to the FDA's authority to regulate human drug compounding.

Chapter 3 – Drug compounding is the process by which a pharmacist combines, mixes, or alters ingredients to create a drug tailored to the medical needs of an individual. An outbreak of fungal meningitis in 2012 linked to contaminated compounded drugs has raised concerns about state and federal oversight of drug compounding. GAO was asked to update its 2003 testimony on drug compounding. Specifically, this report addresses (1) the status of FDA's authority to oversee drug compounding, and the gaps, if any, between state and federal authority; (2) how FDA has used its data and authority to oversee drug compounding; and (3) the actions taken or planned by states or national pharmacy organizations to improve oversight of drug compounding. GAO reviewed relevant statutes and guidance; reviewed FDA data; and interviewed officials from FDA, national pharmacy organizations, and four states with varied geography, population, and pharmacy regulations.

Chapter 4 – Statement of Janet Woodcock, Director, Center for Drug Evaluation and Research, Food and Drug Administration.

Chapter 5 – Testimony of Scott Gottlieb, Resident Fellow, The American Enterprise Institute.

Chapter 6 – Testimony of Joe Harminson, Owner of DFW Prescriptions, on behalf of the National Community Pharmacists Association. Hearing on "Examining Drug Compounding", dated May 23, 2013.

In: Drug Compounding
Editor: Martti Bram
ISBN: 978-1-63117-360-8

Chapter 1

COMPOUNDED DRUGS*

Judith M. Glassgold

SUMMARY

Compounding has been traditionally defined as a process where a pharmacist or a physician combines, mixes, or alters ingredients to create a medication tailored to the needs of an individual patient. Traditionally compounded drugs (CDs) are made in response to an individual prescription from a licensed health provider in the context of a pharmacist's and health care professional's relationship with a specific patient.

Some have suggested that certain activities not traditionally associated with compounding be considered compounding. Such activities include the large-scale production of drugs to ease certain drug shortages, to meet outsourcing needs of hospitals, and to supply physician-administered drugs. Non-traditional compounding may include (1) the production and shipping of large volume of drugs across state lines; (2) production of drugs that are copies of FDA-approved commercially available drugs; (3) provision of CD without a prescription for an individual patient to receive a compounded version and outside of a professional relationship; and (4) production of products to third parties, such as hospitals, clinics, physician offices, and home health providers. These activities could be considered more akin to manufacturing than

* This is an edited, reformatted and augmented version of a Congressional Research Service publication, CRS Report for Congress R43082, prepared for Members and Committees of Congress, from www.crs.gov, dated June 3, 2013.

traditional compounding, which is considered part of the traditional practice of pharmacy.

Adverse events involving contaminated compounded drugs have drawn attention to the growing use of non-traditionally compounded drugs in health care delivery. Shortages of sterile generic drugs and hospital outsourcing are cited as causes of increased numbers of CDs produced by nontraditional compounders. Efforts to assess the risks and benefits of CDs on public health and safety are complicated by the lack of publicly available information, including the absence of a federal adverse event reporting requirement, and the lack of information about the number of drugs compounded, the types of drugs compounded, and the number of businesses in this market.

Policymakers have raised questions regarding how best to improve the safety of CDs while maintaining patient access to needed medications. Drug compounding has historically been the focus of state governments through their regulation of pharmacies. Recently questions have arisen regarding the extent to which the federal government can regulate the practice of compounding through the Federal Food, Drug, and Cosmetic Act (FFDCA). Policy discussions include proposals to clarify federal oversight of high-risk activities and products, to improve federal and state coordination, and to increase use of existing federal authorities.

This report provides background information on CDs and non-traditional compounding pharmacies relevant to policy discussions. This includes an overview of the 2012 fungal meningitis outbreak, recent safety alerts and recalls of compounded drugs, definitions of traditional compounding and non-traditional compounding, information on the CDs produced and by whom, information on the demand for non-traditional compounding, including the role of shortages of sterile injectable drugs, hospital out-sourcing, and patient and provider demand, and information on adverse events involving compounded drugs.

INTRODUCTION

In September 2012, the Centers for Disease Control and Prevention (CDC), the Food and Drug Administration (FDA), the Tennessee Department of Health, and other state health departments[1] began investigating a rare, non-contagious outbreak of fungal meningitis. [2] As of June 3, 2013, 20 states had reported 745 infections (including fungal meningitis and other conditions),[3] and 58 deaths were traced to injections of contaminated, preservative-free methylprednisone acetate produced by the New England Compounding Center (NECC). NECC, which self-identified as a compounding pharmacy – not a manufacturer – and was licensed by the state of Massachusetts, produced large volumes of drugs that were shipped across state lines to health care providers.[4] Unlike traditional pharmacy practices, NECC produced drugs without individual prescriptions and made copies of existing commercially-manufactured drugs.[5]

These serious adverse events[6] drew attention to compounded drugs (CDs).[7] Six congressional hearings were held in 2012-2013 to understand the factors that led to these adverse events and ways to prevent future such incidents; these hearings are listed in *Appendix B*.[8] In these hearings Members of Congress and stakeholders raised questions regarding how best to improve the safety of CDs while maintaining patient access to needed drugs.

Issues raised at these hearings include the following: (1) what are CDs; (2) how are CDs made and by whom; (3) what is the role of CDs in health care delivery; (4) what are the federal and state roles in oversight of CDs; (5) how safe are CDs, and (6) what steps could be taken to prevent adverse events from CDs.

This report provides background information about these issues that may be used to inform the policy discussion as Congress considers legislation. This report focuses on (1) available background information on CDs and compounding pharmacies; (2) changes in the role of CDs in healthcare delivery; (3) factors leading to an increase of compounding; (4) safety of CDs, including a table of selected publicly available adverse events; and (5) a brief summary of policy issues raised to date. This report includes material on CDs for human patients and does not include a discussion of veterinary drug compounding or the compounding of dietary supplements.

Issues of public health and safety of CDs are tied to the regulation and oversight of CDs. This report includes brief information on federal, state, and professional efforts to increase the safety of CDs.

BACKGROUND

Compounding has been traditionally defined as a process where a pharmacist or a physician combines, mixes, or alters ingredients to create a medication tailored to the needs of an individual patient. Traditionally CDs are made in response to an individual prescription from a licensed health provider in the context of a pharmacist's and health care provider's professional relationship with a specific patient. CDs provide alternatives to standard commercially-manufactured drugs when such drugs do not meet the unique medical needs of a patient (e.g., due to a need for an allergen-free drug, weight-based dosing, or alternate modes of delivery), or are unavailable due to discontinuation, unavailability, or shortages. Shortages of sterile generic drugs and hospital outsourcing are cited as causes of increased the reliance of health care providers on CDs.[9]

Some have suggested that certain activities not traditionally associated with compounding be considered compounding. Such activities include the large-scale production of drugs to ease certain drug shortages, to meet outsourcing needs of hospitals, and to supply physician-administered drugs. Non-traditional compounding may include (1) the production and shipping of large volume of drugs across state lines; (2) production of drugs that are copies of FDA-approved commercially available drugs; (3) production of drugs outside of a personal relationship with a patient and without a prescription for an individual patient to receive a compounded version; and (4) providing products to third parties, such as hospitals, clinics, physician offices, and home health providers. These activities may be considered more akin to manufacturing than traditional compounding, which is considered part of the traditional practice of pharmacy. In this report, references to these types of activities will be called "non-traditional compounding." This report will be updated as necessary.

Health Concerns Involving CDs

Background

Adverse events stemming from CDs in 2012 are the starting point for the current policy debate about existing regulatory oversight of CDs.[10] The 2012 fungal meningitis outbreak was triggered by contaminated sterile CDs, injectable methylprednisolone, and was the worst recorded adverse event involving CDs,[11] with news reports indicating that up to 14,000 individuals were exposed to this product.[12] Contaminated sterile drugs pose the most serious threats to human health, and can cause death.[13] Details on this event are listed in the following text box.[14]

Fall 2012 Fungal Meningitis Events

- September 26, 2012, NECC recalls three lots of methylprednisolone acetate, an injectable steroid.

- October 4, 2012, the FDA verified that NECC, a compounding center in Massachusetts, was the source of the contaminated compounded injectable methylprednisolone.[15]
- October 6, 2012, NECC recalled all compounded products from its Framingham, MA facility.[16] The FDA urges health care providers to follow up with patients who received injectable and ophthalmic products.
- October 31, 2012, Ameridose, a company associated with NECC, recalled all unexpired products in circulation.

Source: CDC "Related Drug Recalls" http://www.cdc.gov/hai/outbreaks/current situation/archive.html, accessed May 6, 2012.

The safety of CDs has been a concern of Congress for over two decades due to the expansion of non-traditional compounding.[17] Potential safety risks for CDs include problems with *potency* (i.e., the dosage is inaccurate, either too strong or too weak), *purity* (e.g., the drug contains other chemicals that could be harmful), and *contamination* (the drug is contaminated with a bacteria, fungus, or virus).[18]

The FDA conducted surveys in 2001 and 2006 to assess identity, strength, quality and purity issues for CDs. [19] In a non-random survey of compounded drugs available over the Internet, about one-third (33%) failed analytic testing, mostly regarding potency or uniformity of dosage. In these surveys, the rates of analytic testing failures for compounded drugs were higher than those for commercially-available drugs, where only 2% of drugs failed analytic testing.[20] There is no specific federal or state requirement that an individual CD be tested for potency, purity, and sterility prior to being sold or administered.[21] The compounder of a product may voluntarily perform such tests along with other quality control processes.[22]

Safety issues with CDs also have been found by state pharmacy boards. [23] Certain states have started testing a certain percentage of compounded drugs for non-disciplinary purposes. For example, the State of Missouri Board of Pharmacy initiated a testing program in 2003 for compounded drugs and each year tests a certain number of finished products.[24] Over the course of the testing program, 15% - 25% of the CDs were found to have problems with drug potency, ranging from a sub-potent drug with 0%—no active ingredient present—to a super-potent drug with almost 400% of the prescribed dosage. An inaccurate dose may present a risk of harm to the patient through a risk of toxicity (super-potent) or the risk of ineffective treatment (sub-potency) (see for example, *Table C-1*, years 2010, 2007).[25]

The lack of resources to carry out testing of CDs appears to be a problem in several states.[26] For example, a newspaper reported that Texas passed a law to provide for inspections of compounding pharmacies, but did not authorize funds for such purposes until 2007; once funded, testing dropped by two-thirds in 2012 compared to 2010 due to state budget cuts.[27]

Adverse Event Reporting

There is no federal requirement for producers of CDs to report adverse events, so the actual number of individuals harmed by CDs is unknown.[28] Policymakers have had concerns with CDs[29] that date back almost two decades;[30] these include reports of contamination of products that should be sterile, sub- or super-potent dosages, and impurities.[31]

Table C-1 provides a selected compilation of publicly available reports of adverse events involving CDs and other compounded medical products with details about the date, the number of states affected, the number of people affected, mortality (if any), drug involved, condition treated, and other characteristics, such as whether the product was shipped across state lines or was an off-label use.[32] The vast majority of these adverse events involve sterile compounded products.[33] Sterile compounded products include injectable drugs, IV-delivered drugs and solutions, inhalation drugs, and parenteral nutrition that are administered directly into the body and must be sterile to assure patient safety.[34]

There is no specific federal requirement for the reporting of adverse events with CDs; so that this information is by nature selective and cannot be used to draw inferences about the overall risks of CDs. Reports of incidents with CDs that do not rise to adverse events are excluded from the table.[35] *Table C-1* also includes other characteristics of CDs, including where it was evident that CDs were shipped across state lines, an element of non-traditional compounding and high-volume facilities, whether CD were prescribed for off-label uses, and whether a drug shortage was in effect. For example, a shortage of generic preservative-free methylprednisolone was reported by some sources prior to the 2012 fungal meningitis outbreak, which was caused by compounded versions of that drug.[36]

The 2012 fungal meningitis outbreak led to greater scrutiny by federal and state authorities of sterile CDs.[37] In 2013, FDA and state authorities inspected certain facilities that produce sterile CDs and found a variety of safety concerns.[38] Later, some, but not all, of these compounders issued product recalls due to sterility concerns.[39]

The next adverse event linked to a nontraditional compounding pharmacy occurred on May 24, 2013, when the FDA reported infections linked to contaminated sterile injectables; on May 28, 2013, the compounder recalled certain sterile products.[40] Recalls of sterile CDs for 2013 are listed in the following text box.[41]

2013 Manufacturer Recalls of Sterile CDs as of May 31, 2013

- On May 29, 2013, Lowlite Investments (doing business as Olympia Pharmacy) announced a voluntary multi-state recall of all sterile drug products supplied to patients and offices of licensed medical professionals with a use by date of September 25, 2013, or earlier. The recall is being initiated due to concerns associated with prior quality control procedures that impacted sterility assurance. No adverse events had been reported as of the date of the recall.[42]
- On May 24, 2013, the FDA posted a notice that the CDC, the Tennessee Board of Pharmacy and the FDA were investigating reports of seven adverse events associated with compounded preservative-free methylprednisolone injections compounded by Main Street Family Pharmacy, LLC. These reports link infections, one of which is fungal in nature.[43] On May 28, 2013, Main Street Family Pharmacy, LLC recalled all sterile products with a use by date on or before November 20, 2013.[44]
- On May 15, 2013, the FDA announced that Pentec Health, Inc. initiated a recall of nutritional prescriptions for renal patient due to a lack of sterility assurance. No adverse events had been reported as of the date of recall.[45]
- On May 6, 2013, the FDA alerted health care providers of concerns regarding sterility assurance for sterile drugs produced and distributed by the Compounding Shop. The FDA reports that the Compounding Shop is in the process of recalling products. No adverse events had been reported as of the date of recall.[46]
- On April 22, 2013, Nora Apothecary and Alternative Medicine recalled all lots of sterile compounded products produced on or before April 19, 2013 due to the lack of sterility assurance and concerns associated with the quality control processes. No adverse events had been reported as of the date of recall.[47]
- On April 17, 2013, Balanced Solutions Compounding Pharmacy

(Balanced Solutions), a division of Axium Healthcare Pharmacy, Inc., of Lake Mary, FL, recalled all lots of its sterile non-expired drug products due to a lack of sterility assurances associated with the quality control processes. No adverse incidents had been reported as of the date of recall.[48]

- On April 15, 2013, NuVision Pharmacy recalled all lots of all compounded lyophilized products due to sterility assurance concerns. No adverse events had been reported as of the date of recall.[49] On May 18, 2013, the FDA expanded its alert to health care providers to all sterile drug products made and distributed by NuVision.[50]
- On April 15, 2013, ApothéCure, Inc. recalled all lots of all sterile products compounded, repackaged, and distributed by Apothécure, Inc. due to sterility assurance concerns. No adverse events had been reported as of the date of recall.[51]
- On April 05, 2013, Green Valley Drugs recalled all lots of all sterile products compounded, repackaged, and distributed by the firm due to quality control concerns. No adverse events had been reported as of the date of recall.[52]
- On March 25, 2013, state regulators halted production of sterile products made by Pallimed, a compounding pharmacy, and requested a recall of all sterile products.[53] Pallimed issued such a recall March 26, 2013. No adverse events had been reported as of the date of recall.[54]
- On March 20, 2013, Clinical Specialties Compounding Pharmacy recalled all sterile products repackaged and distributed due to the company's lack of confidence in product sterility.[55] This followed a recall on March 18, 2013, of Avastin compounded for ophthalmic use. No adverse events had been reported as of the date of recall.[56]
- On March 17, 2013, Med Prep recalled all lots of its compounded drugs due to mold contamination.[57] This followed the recall of a single product line on March 16, 2013. No adverse events had been reported as of the date of recall.[58]

Traditional Compounding

Traditional compounding is a process where a pharmacist or a physician "combines, mixes, or alters ingredients to create a medication tailored to the needs of an individual patient"[59] in response to a prescription from a health care provider. CDs can include different formulations of drugs (e.g., liquid instead of tablet), doses, and certain ingredients (e.g., allergen-free, dye-free).

[60] This report will use the phrase "traditional compounding" to reference the historical use of the term compounding.

CDs can provide patients drugs tailored to their individual health needs. The benefits of traditional compounding include (1) providing individualized drugs when commercially-produced drugs do not meet the health requirements of an individual patient; and (2) maintaining access to certain prescription drugs that are not commercially available due to shortages, unavailability, or discontinuation, among other factors.[61]

The number of CDs made cannot be determined due to the lack of publicly available information.[62] Currently no federal reporting requirement exists for producers of CDs with respect to their compounding activities.[63] The most recent attempt to assess the number of CDs was through a survey commissioned by the FDA in 2001. This report estimated that 650 pharmacies filled about 13 million prescriptions for compounded prescription drugs per year.[64] Some stakeholders estimate that anywhere from 1-5% of all prescriptions filled annually are for CDs,[65] but the basis of this information cannot be verified. [66]

There is also no publicly available information on the types of CDs made, for instance, the percentage of CDs that include dosage, formulation, or ingredient alterations, or that are produced in response to shortages of commercially-manufactured drugs. The lack of information on the current scope of compounding presents challenges for public health authorities and policy makers.

Pharmacists, or technicians supervised by a licensed pharmacist, and physicians can produce CDs.[67] Compounding is part of the standard practice of pharmacy and is within the scope of state licensure of pharmacists and pharmacies.[68] The number of pharmacists engaged in compounding on a regular basis is difficult to evaluate due to a lack of publicly available information.[69] The most recent attempt to survey pharmacists, commissioned by the FDA, found that the majority of compounded prescriptions are filled by a small number of pharmacies, and for some, CDs are the majority of their business.[70] Others provide different estimates. Janet Woodcock, Director of the FDA Center for Drug Evaluation and Research (CDER), stated in a recent interview that 28,000 pharmacies compound drugs nationwide.[71] The American Pharmacists Association (APhA), a trade association of pharmacists, reports that there are 7,500 pharmacies in the United States that specialize in compounding.[72] The International Academy of Compounding Pharmacies, a trade association representing the compounding profession, has 2,700 members.[73] As of January, 2013 there were 163 pharmacies in the United

States accredited by the Pharmacy Compounding Accreditation Board, which offers a voluntary accreditation process for compounding pharmacies.[74]

Existing sources of publicly available information on specific CD products include those listed by compounding pharmacies on their websites,[75] products described by professional associations,[76] products mentioned in scientific journals, and on CDC and FDA websites due to warning and other notices.[77]

These CDs include, among others, drugs for: pain management (including alternate delivery, combined medications, dosage variations), hormone replacement therapies for women (including bioidentical hormones) and men (e.g., testosterone), men's and women's health, sports medicine, weight-loss, dental care, veterinary care, pediatric patients, and hospice care.[78] Some compounded products include items advertised as treatments for Autism/ADHD,[79] "adrenal fatigue,"[80] or fat-elimination;[81] the FDA and others have raised questions regarding these claims.[82]

Non-Traditional Compounding

As noted earlier, some enterprises have engaged in certain activities not traditionally associated with compounding, but have asserted that these activities should be considered compounding.[83]

Such activities include the large-scale production of drugs to ease certain drug shortages, to meet outsourcing needs of hospitals and to supply physician-administered drugs.[84] Non-traditional compounders make a variety of products, including sterile injectables, parenteral nutrition, and drugs on the FDA shortage list.[85] Sterile injectable CDs include epidurals (for childbirth and pain management), nerve-blocking agents, drugs for pain management, and antibiotics.[86] Individuals might receive these products in a hospital, doctor's office, or other medical facility as a medication, an IV solution or nutrition.

Some non-traditional compounders have large numbers of customers. For example, PharMedium, a large scale compounder, reported 2,300 hospital customers for a variety of compounded products.[87] NECC, the compounder involved in the fungal meningitis outbreak of 2012, was listed on a FDA website as having over 20,000 customers, including physicians, clinics, and hospitals.[88]

EXISTING REGULATORY OVERSIGHT

Drug compounding has historically been the focus of state governments through their regulation of pharmacies. Recently questions have arisen regarding the extent the federal government can regulate the practice of compounding through the FFDCA. This section discusses federal and state authorities, as well as industry self-regulation.

Federal Authorities[89]

Federal authority over compounding largely stems from the Federal Food Drug and Cosmetics Act (FFDCA), enacted in 1938, and its subsequent amendments, including the Food and Drug Administration Modernization Act (FDAMA) of 1997, which added compounding-specific provisions to the FFDCA in Section 503A. Litigation over Section 503A's advertising provisions has created doubt, however, over the legal effect of FDAMA's compounding provisions.[90]

The precise limit to federal authority with respect to drug compounding remains uncertain as the federal authority to regulate traditional drug compounding has been discussed by very few courts, and each court that has approached the issue did so from a unique factual setting that colored the eventual outcome of the case.[91] Courts appear to agree that the federal government can regulate compounding activity that is akin to manufacturing (i.e., non-traditional compounding), and courts have afforded deference to the FDA's interpretation of when a compounder is acting like a manufacturer, which appears to be within the FDA's discretion.[92] However, there is not a bright-line distinction between behaviors that are "akin to manufacturing" and those of a traditional compounding pharmacy. As a result, uncertainty remains regarding the possible limits to the FDA's current authority to regulate traditional compounding practices.

Even assuming that FDA has the authority to regulate traditional compounding, as a matter of policy, the FDA has generally declined to test the current limits of its authority to regulate compounding, preferring instead to defer to state governments with respect to the regulation of "traditional compounding."[93]

State Authorities

Traditional compounding is a component of the practice of pharmacy and has typically been regulated by the states as "part of their regulation of pharmacies"[94] and the licensing of pharmacists as health care professionals.[95] There is great variety in existing state legislation addressing CDs.[96] Certain states have passed new laws, or are considering revisions of laws and regulations for compounding pharmacies, in part due to recent events.[97] The National Association of Boards of Pharmacies (NABP) has listed summaries of approved and proposed state changes to permitted compounding practices.[98]

State boards of pharmacy evaluate pharmacists and pharmacies on compounding practices and facilities.[99] Compounding from bulk ingredients is generally an approved part of pharmacy practice,[100] with some states requiring all licensed pharmacies to offer compounding services.[101]

Some states follow NABP model language and permit a pharmacist to compound drugs to patients only upon receipt of a valid prescription from a doctor or other medical practitioner licensed to prescribe medication.[102] Some states require a special license for compounding sterile medications, which requires special facilities and adherence to sterile methods.[103] Other states license a separate class of pharmacy facility that produces drugs for pharmacies or other providers, such as central fill pharmacies.[104] Finally, some states permit pharmacies to make exact copies of commercial products in response to discontinued products or drug shortages. [105]

Industry Self-Regulation

Professional programs in pharmacy are accredited and pharmacists generally receive formal education and professional training with respect to the practice of compounding drugs.[106] Pharmacists can participate in a voluntary accreditation process for compounding established by professional pharmacy organizations, and the U.S. Pharmacopeial Convention (USP). [107] As of December 2012, 163 facilities nationwide have this accreditation.[108]

Professional standards and guidelines for CDs are established by the USP in published standards: Chapter 797 "Pharmaceutical Compounding – Sterile Preparations" for sterile products and Chapter 795 "Pharmaceutical Compounding – Non-Sterile Preparations." USP Standard 797 includes standards for facilities, procedures, and staff in order to produce safe sterile drugs, such as sterilizing equipment, a sterile clean room, special ventilation, and decontamination processes.[109]

Not all pharmacies or compounders adhere to these USP standards and these standards, unless required by state law, are voluntary.[110] To date, 20 states have laws that require full adherence to USP Standard 797.[111]

USP standards are designed for pharmacy compounding and may not be suitable for large-scale production of CDs.[112] Commercial production of drugs is addressed by the current good manufacturing practices (cGMP) required by Section 501 of the FFDCA for commercial manufacturers; cGMP requires certain manufacturing practices as well as adverse event reporting.[113]

GROWTH OF NON-TRADITIONAL COMPOUNDING

Some believe that the number and types of CDs and other products (IV and parenteral nutrition) are increasing,[114] coinciding with increasing demand for certain compounded products[115] due to a variety of reasons, including (1) an increase in hospital outsourcing of CDs; (2) drug shortages, unavailability, and discontinuation of FDA-approved drugs;[116] (3) interest in individualized products by physicians and consumers; and (4) an increased interest by pharmacists in new markets.[117]

As noted earlier, the exact number of business facilities engaged in non-traditional compounding is unclear.[118] In 2013, the FDA inspected non-traditional compounding facilities that were engaged in sterile compounding and lists 39 facilities that it inspected located around the country.[119] Some of these facilities, such as Central Admixture Pharmacy Services and PharMEDium Services have multiple locations. Press and other sources indicate growth of centralized compounding facilities that provide outsourcing and related activities to pharmacies and hospitals.[120] Some of these compounding facilities include compounding pharmacies, central fill pharmacies,[121] and outsourcing pharmacies.[122] Some states, but not all, permit certain types of consolidated services, such as "shared services" or "central fill IV pharmacies,"[123] which make products for distribution among a variety of providers. For example, Med Prep Consulting, Inc. lists itself as a state-licensed central fill pharmacy and provides products to other pharmacies.[124]

Hospital Compounding and Outsourcing

Hospitals commonly compound drugs, IV solutions, and IV nutrition. For example, children's hospitals compound a variety of products such as pediatric dosages or products that are not commercially available.[125] One source reports that increases in use of drugs dosed by weight,[126] rather than in commercially-available dosing, and the expansion of treatment of disorders that require personalized dosing have led to a growth of hospital-based compounding.[127]

Trends in health care include increasing hospital consolidation and integration of hospitals,[128] leading to consolidated purchasing and centralized production, including the production of CDs.[129] For example, the Cleveland Clinic Health System, a network of 10 hospitals and 15 pharmacies, reported that in 2012, approximately 870,000 doses were compounded at its central facility.[130] Cleveland Clinic reported that 56% of its products were compounded for the needs of specific patients;[131] 44% were made in anticipation of patient needs in a large hospital, such as the preparation of syringes used in the operating room, epidurals, narcotic infusions, doses not commercially available, and medications that were unavailable due to drug shortages.[132] Smaller facilities in rural areas may increase the outsourcing of CDs due to need for specialty intravenous products without the facilities to produce such products.[133] Reductions in staff or insufficient staff or facilities to continue compounding; streamlining workflow; and cost savings may also be factors related to outsourcing by facilities.[134]

As noted earlier, there is limited information on the numbers of outsourced compounded products, as the records of compounding entities are not publicly reported. However, a 2013 report of the Office of the Inspector General (OIG) of the Department of Health and Human Services (HHS) on outsourcing of sterile products by hospitals found that 25% used "high-risk" sterile products, those made from non-sterile ingredients, while 92 % of hospitals used compounded sterile products that were not "high-risk".[135] The reasons hospitals provided for outsourcing sterile compounded products include drug shortages and their lack of capacity to produce products that remained stable over time and thus had a long shelf-life. Stability and extended shelf-life permit hospitals to store products for use as patient needs emerge.

Shortages were cited as a reason for outsourcing by 62% of hospitals, as were stability (69%) and extended shelf-life (62%).[136]

The Role of Drug Shortages in CD Demand

Shortages of Generic Injectable Drugs

Shortages of commercially-available drugs, especially shortages of generic sterile products, play a central role in the increased demand for CDs.[137] The drug shortages may be temporary or permanent and are due to a variety of factors including voluntary discontinuation of products, supply chain problems, and production issues, including safety problems at commercial manufacturers.[138] Certain compounders advertise their ability to fill certain back-ordered drugs or those in short supply on their websites.[139] Shortages of commercially-manufactured drug are predicted to continue, leading to continued demand for certain compounded products.[140]

Physicians, hospitals, and other health care providers may turn to compounders to meet a time-sensitive need when specific drugs may be temporarily unavailable.[141] A 2013 report by the Office of the Inspector General (OIG) of the Department of Health and Human Services (HHS) surveyed hospitals participating in Medicare and found that many hospitals turn to compounding pharmacies to provide drugs to maintain supply due to shortages of commercially-manufactured FDA-approved drugs. According to the OIG report, 68% of hospitals indicated that they sought a CD due to a drug shortage.[142]

The FDA and other safety advocates are concerned because reportedly 73% of drug shortages are for sterile injectable generic drugs, which are some of the most difficult drugs to compound safely.[143] Several generic commercial manufacturers have struggled with manufacturing problems that have led to interruptions in supply of sterile generic drugs.[144] For example, as of May 15, 2013, a major generic manufacturer in this business sector, Hospira, has recalled eight different sterile injectable drugs for 2012 and 2013.[145] An alternative to sterile injectable CDs and generics are brand-name sterile injectables. These are less likely to be in short supply or suffer from quality problems;[146] however, brand-name sterile drugs usually cost more than generic or compounded products.[147]

Shortages of CDs

Recalls of products from compounding pharmacies may also exacerbate drug shortages.[148] Ameridose and NECC ended production of certain sterile drugs in 2012-2013 due to problems with sterility, and these drugs were already in short supply.[149] In 2013, compounders recalled certain products produced at these facilities;[150] some of these products were drugs listed on the

FDA shortages website. For example, drugs recalled by Med Prep in March 2013 include drugs on the FDA Current Drug Shortage Index.[151]

CD shortages heighten problems of patient access to commercially-manufactured generic drugs when there are shortages. *Table 1* details the perceptions of hospitals about the effect of disruptions in supply of sterile products from compounding pharmacies. Almost 50% of respondents perceived that health care delivery would be seriously impacted, while 11.5% perceived that the effect on patient health would be life-threatening.

Table 1. Hospital Beliefs About The Effect of Shortages of Compounded Sterile Products on Patient Care and Health Care Delivery

Perceived Level of Risk to Patients/Disruption of Care	Percentage of Hospitals
Life Threatening/Major Disruptions	11.5
Not Life Threatening/Great Impact	48.1
Little Impact/Inconvenience	16.6
No Impact at All	23.8

Source: Adapted by CRS from Office of Inspector General, Department of Health and Human Services, Memorandum Report; "High Risk Compounded Sterile Preparations and Outsourcing by Hospitals that Use Them" OEI-01-13-00150, p. 14.

Other Sources of Demand for Compounded Products

A growth of interest in customized products, including allergen-free drugs, single administration of multiple drugs, and individualized formulations of drugs (such as liquids instead of tablets) may play a role in heightened demand for CDs.[152] The sources of this demand include physician and patient demand as well as changing pharmacist business models. There appears to be an increase in marketing of CDs for treatment of common disorders, such as menopausal symptoms (e.g., "bio-identical" hormones), men's health, and weight loss, which may lead to an increase in demand for these CDs.[153 154]

Pharmacist Business Development

Compounding may provide pharmacists alternatives to expand business growth. Pharmacy publications have emphasized how compounding pharmacists improve their own professional satisfaction through providing more individualized services and increased engagement with patients.[155] This reflects an evolution to business models that expand pharmacist roles in areas of patient care beyond distributing commercially-manufactured products.[156]

A 2012 article in *Business Week* describes drug compounding as a growing business sector, and describes how focusing on compounding can provide a new market niche for community pharmacies.[157] Some of these pharmacies may be exploring new business models due to increased competition with chain pharmacies and retailers to fill prescriptions for commercially-manufactured drugs. This account appears consistent with material on certain compounding pharmacies' websites that describe business development from community pharmacies into a market niche in compounded products (both prescription drugs and dietary supplements).[158]

Provider Demand

Demand may be generated in part by off-label prescribing by physicians for a variety of reasons, including drug prices and shortages. As *Table C-1* indicates, some of the incidents of contamination and adverse events are for CDs prescribed for off-label uses. Off-label prescribing allows physicians flexibility to prescribe medications they feel are necessary for patient health.[159] Off-label use of a CD may present additional, but unknown risks. For example, two common off-label uses of sterile CD are a compounded version of a chemotherapy drug, Avastin, for use to treat macular degeneration, and preservative-free methylprednisolone for back pain.[160] There have been recent adverse events with compounded Avastin, the main appeal of which is its lower price compared to FDA-approved drugs to treat macular degeneration (see *Table C-1*, 2011).[161] Preservative-free methylprednisolone is used to treat back pain (see *Table C-1*, years 2013, 2012, 2002, 2001). Compounded versions of this drug by NECC were the cause of the 2012 fungal meningitis outbreak.[162]

The processes for creating sterile CDs require special equipment, facilities, and personnel training.[163] When compounding exclusively with sterile ingredients, sterility must be maintained in all phases of production; when compounding with non-sterile ingredients, sterility must be achieved for the finished product requiring a sterilization process or related procedure that does not affect product stability. Regulators and industry agree that the highest risk to patient safety is from those sterile products made from non-sterile ingredients.[164]

ISSUES FOR CONSIDERATION

Consumers, pharmacists, pharmacy compounders, hospitals, Congress, and state and federal regulators all have a stake in access to, and safety of, needed drugs. Increasing demand for CDs by patients and providers, drug shortages, consolidation of hospital services and other factors have led to changes in health delivery. The potential risks to public health of product failures have increased as non-traditional compounding has expanded.[165] Given the expansion of sterile compounding, balancing patient access to CDs with patient safety has become more complex.[166] Thus, some stakeholders believe that changes in business trends, such as drug shortages and outsourcing of compounding, must be taken into consideration in considering changes in professional standards and federal and state oversight and regulation of CD.[167]

Three issues have emerged in the congressional hearings about CDs and in legislation introduced in the 112th and 113th Congress (see *Table A-1*): (1) adverse event reporting, (2) labeling, and (3) modifying federal oversight of non-traditional compounding. These issues will be discussed in the following section.

Adverse Event Reporting and Labeling

There is a lack of publically available information on the number and types of adverse events involving compounded drugs, as there is no requirement that compounders report adverse events to federal authorities,[168] and state requirements vary.[169] Adverse event reporting is not required by federal regulators for producers of CDs as it is for prescription, non-prescription drugs, and dietary supplements.[170] Without knowing the total number of compounded products made, as well as the total number of adverse events, it is difficult to ascertain the overall safety of CDs or to understand the benefits and risks of using CDs.

The publicly-available information on CDs is published by public health authorities, FDA inspections of facilities listed on websites, records of state licensing boards, and reports in professional journals documenting adverse events. Adverse events can be voluntarily reported to the FDA MedWatch database, but without mandatory reporting, the completeness of the information cannot be ascertained.[171]

Labeling specifying that a drug or another product is compounded is not a universal requirement.[172] Due to the complexity of the supply chain and the growth of non-traditional compounding, patients and providers may not realize that a drug has been compounded. Unlike traditional compounding where a patient is given a prescription by a physician for a CD, nontraditional CDs are not necessarily identified as compounded.[173] Given the potential benefits and risks of CDs, an argument could be made for providing patients this information as part of informed consent for medical treatment.[174] Informed consent for treatment is an ethical and a legal requirement to ensure that a patient fully understands the potential risks and benefits of a medical procedure.[175] CDs and other compounded solutions pose potential risks and benefits that may be different from commercially-manufactured products. Informed consent is based on a patient's knowledge and understanding of a medical procedure; as most patients assume that drugs are commercially-manufactured, this additional information could be seen as necessary to the ethical pursuit of informed patient consent.[176]

The Federal Role in Oversight

Policymakers have raised questions regarding how best to improve the safety of CDs while maintaining patient access to needed medications, including the need for new legislation and increased accountability. [177] In testimony to Congress, FDA administrators have expressed reservations about non-traditional compounding activities that are akin to manufacturing (i.e., non-traditional compounding) and their potential risks to public safety.[178] The FDA recommends increased federal oversight of sterile compounding and certain other high-risk activities.[179]

Attempts to clarify federal authority over non-traditional compounding is represented in certain elements of bipartisan legislation of the Senate Committee on Health, Education, Labor and Pensions (HELP)[180] and in legislation introduced in the 112th and 113th Congress.[181] These proposals all include increased clarity in the federal oversight role for compounding drugs. For example, a provision in the draft HELP legislation would create new authorities for FDA oversight of "compounding manufacturers" (i.e., non-traditional compounders) (see *Table A1*).[182]

Some Members of Congress argue that new FDA authorities should await better implementation of existing authorities.[183] For example, a House Committee on Energy and Commerce report questions whether a lack of enforcement by FDA and state authorities of certain vendors is an issue.[184] The report cites safety violations at NECC in prior years, which do not appear to have been resolved despite FDA involvement.[185]

Some in the compounding pharmacy industry believe that the current safety issues are isolated to certain vendors and that compounding, in general, is not unsafe.[186] Some compounding associations have reservations about the FDA having new authorities; others support increased FDA oversight.[187] Many acknowledge that compounded health care products have become more complex and health delivery more complicated. In a recent report, the Association of Health-System Pharmacists (AHSP) and American Hospital Association (AHA) noted that there was general support from stakeholders in these associations for (1) FDA oversight of certain nontraditional compounding pharmacies (e.g., providing a CD without a prescription and shipped over state lines); (2) improved communication between state and federal regulators; (3) a list of "do-not-compound" CDs; and (4) improved access to USP compounding monographs that provide guidance to compounders on making certain CDs.[188]

Appendix A. Legislation Introduced in the 113th Congress Affecting Drug Compounding

The following table summarizes selected provisions of the two pieces of legislation on compounding introduced to date in the 113th Congress. It includes provisions that address issues discussed in this report, but it does not provide a full summary of the legislation.

Table A-1. Selected Issues in S. 959 and H.R. 2186

	S. 959	H.R. 2186
	Bill Status: Committee Actions: Ordered	
Issues	to be Reported	Bills Status: Introduced
Adverse Event Reporting	Yes	Yes
Federal Authorities	(1) Would clarify that a "new drug" (Section 201(p) of the FFDCA) includes compounded human drugs; (2) contains specific provisions regarding "traditional	Provides that certain adulteration and misbranding provisions of the FFDCA and the "new drug" provisions of the FFDCA do not apply to certain compounded drugs.

	S. 959	H.R. 2186
	Bill Status: Committee Actions: Ordered	
Issues	to be Reported	Bills Status: Introduced
	compounders" and "compounding manufacturers."	
Federal Registration of Certain Compounders	Yes	Yes
Labeling	Would require specific labeling as compounded drug, among other requirements. Drug would be considered misbranded (and would be subject to penalties) under FFDCA if not so labeled.	Would require specific labeling as compounded drug, among other requirements. Drug would be considered misbranded (and would be subject to penalties) under FFDCA if not so labeled.
Registration of Compounders	Yes, fee would be required to off-set costs of inspection and oversight.	Yes, fee would be required to off-set costs of inspection and oversight.
Shortages	Would permit copies of FDA-approved drugs during verified shortages.	Would permit copies of FDA-approved drugs during verified shortages.
Special Rules for Sterile Compounding	Yes, would clarify FDA oversight regarding sterile manufacturers who ship across state lines, and would create new manufacturing standards for these products.	Yes, would create new manufacturing standards for "high-risk" sterile compounding.

Source: CRS review of legislation: S. 959 ; H.R. 2186.

Note: FFDCA is the Federal Food, Drug, and Cosmetic Act as amended (21 U.S.C. § 301 et seq.).

APPENDIX B. CONGRESSIONAL HEARINGS ON CDS 2012-2013 (IN REVERSE CHRONOLOGICAL ORDER)

- "Examining Drug Compounding," hearing of the Subcommittee on Health of the Committee on Energy and Commerce, U.S. House of Representatives, May 23, 2013.
- Executive Session, S. 959 Pharmaceutical Compounding Quality and Accountability Act, hearing of the Committee on Health, Education, Labor, and Pensions, U.S. Senate, May 22, 2013. Ordered to be reported with an amendment in the nature of a substitute favorably.

- "Pharmaceutical Compounding: Proposed Legislative Solution," hearing of the Committee on Health, Education, Labor, and Pensions, U.S. Senate, May 9, 2013.
- "A Continuing Investigation into the Fungal Meningitis Outbreak and Whether It Could Have Been Prevented?", hearing of the Subcommittee on Oversight and Investigations, Committee on Energy and Commerce, U.S. House of Representatives, April 26, 2013.
- "Pharmacy Compounding: Implications of the 2012 Meningitis Outbreak," hearing of the Committee on Health, Education, Labor, and Pensions, U.S. Senate, November 15, 2012.
- "The Fungal Meningitis Outbreak: Could It Have Been Prevented?", hearing of the Subcommittee on Oversight and Investigations, Committee on Energy and Commerce, U.S. House of Representatives, November 14, 2012.

Source: House Committee on Energy and Commerce: http://energycommerce.house.gov/hearings; Senate Committee on Health, Education, Labor and Pensions: http://www.help.senate.gov/hearings/.

APPENDIX C. SELECTED ADVERSE EVENTS INVOLVING COMPOUNDED DRUGS AND SOLUTIONS

Table C-1. Adverse Events 2001-May 30, 2013

Date	# States Affected	Repor-ted Cases	Repor-ted Deaths	Adverse Events	Drug Issue	Condition/ Disease Treated	Product	Other Characteristics
2013	13	7	0	Skin abscess, including fungal infection	Contamina-tion[a]	Lumbar and other back pain	Lumbar and other back pain	Off-label use, shipped across state lines
2012	20	741	55	Fungal meningitis and other infections[b]	Fungal contamina-tion	Lumbar and other back pain	Lumbar and other back pain	Off-label use, shipped across state lines, drug shortage
2012 -2011	6	33	NA	Fungal eye infection, 23 cases of partial to	Fungal contamina-tion	Eye surgery	Eye injections, Brilliant B retinal dye	Shipped across state lines

				severe vision loss[c]			and triamcinolone	
2011	2	21	NA	Bacterial eye infection, one case of meningitis and encephalitis; four cases of loss of eyesight, 3 cases eye removal[d]	Bacterial contamination	Macular degeneration	Eye injections: Intravitreal use of bevacizuma b (Avastin) injections	Off-label use, shipped across state lines
2011	1	5	NA	Blindness[e]	Lack of purity – presence of another medication	Macular degeneration	Eye injections: intravitreal use of bevacizuma b (Avastin) injections	Off-label use
2011	1	19	9	Bacterial bloodstream infection[f]	Bacterial contamination	Nutrition	Parenteral nutrition solution	Drug Shortage
2010	1	1	1	Fatal overdose[g]	Super-potent dosage	IV solution	Sodium chloride	- -
2007	2	3	3	Fatal overdose[h]	Super-potent dosage	Back pain	Colchicine	Off-label use
2007	2	8	NA	Bacterial bloodstream infection[i]	Bacterial contamination	Pain control	IV-solution, fentanyl	Shipped across state lines
2007	1	1	1	Drug toxicity[j]	Drug Stability/ Age	Chronic airway infection	Antibiotic administered by nebulizer	Off-label use
2006-2004	6	80	NA	Bacterial bloodstream infection[k]	Bacterial contamination	IV flush, reduction of blood clots	IV solution heparin/ saline	Shipped across state lines
2006	1	1	1 (pediatric)	Fatal overdose[l]	Super-potent dosage	Cancer	Chemotherapy infusion	- -
2006	1	1	1 (pediatric)	Fatal overdose[m]	Super-potent dosage	Nutrition	Parenteral nutrition	- -
2005	Unavailable*e*	2	NA	Bacterial bloodstream infection[n]	Bacterial Contamination	IV flush	Preservative-free heparinized saline	- -

Table C-1. (Continued)

Date	# States Affected	Repor -ted Cases	Repor- ted Deaths	Adverse Events	Drug Issue	Condition/ Disease Treated	Product	Other Characteristics
2005	1	5	3	Systemic inflamma- tory response syndrome[o]	Contamina- tion	Cardiac conditions	Health infusion, cardioplegia	Shipped across state lines
2005	2	6	NA	Bacterial eye infection, partial or complete loss of vision, 2 eye removals[p]	Bacterial contamina- tion	Assess- ment of eye conditions	Trypan blue – eye stain	Shipped across state lines
2005	5	18	NA	Bacterial bloodstream infection[q]	Bacterial contamina- tion	IV solution	Magnesium sulfate	Shipped across state lines
2004	1	2	NA	Bacterial bloodstream infection (pediatric)[r]	Bacterial contamina- tion	IV flush syringes	Heparin/van comycin, hemophilia	Shipped across state lines
2004	5	64	NA	Bacterial bloodstream infection[s]	Bacterial contamina- tion	IV flush syringes	Heparin/- saline	Shipped across state lines
2004	1	16	NA	Hepatitis C infection[t]	Contaminate d with Hepatitis C virus	Diagnosis of cardiac conditions	Radio- isotope use in cardiac stress tests	- -
2002	1	5	1	Fungal meningitis[u]	Fungal contamina- tion	Back pain	Preservative -free methylpredn isolone acetate injections	Off-label use, drug shortage
2001	1	11	3	Bacterial meningitis, epidural abscess, injected joints and spine[v]	Fungal contamina- tion	Back pain, joint pain	Preservative -free betametha- sone injection	Off-label use, drug shortage
2001	1	4 (pedi atric)	NA	Bacterial meningitis, other infections[w]	Bacterial contamina- tion	Gastric reflux	IV Ranitidine	- -

Source: This list has two sources (1) a CRS literature search of medical and scientific databases such as Medline and PubMed with search terms included "drug compounding," and "adverse effects," "quality control," "risk assessment," "drug contamination," "disease outbreaks," "complications," "administration and dosage," "fatal outcome," and "medication errors." These selected adverse events resulted in reported patient illness and/or death. This is list is not comprehensive as not all adverse effects of compounded medications may be reported to federal and state authorities or result in published articles; (2) Pew Charitable Trust compilation of adverse events associated with compounded medications (200 1 - present), Appendix B of Summary of Stakeholder Meeting, Pharmacy Sterile Compounding Summit. Available at http://www.ashp.org/compounding% 20summit, accessed April 18, 2012. The CRS and Pew Trust lists overlap except for two adverse events that are included only in this report; these two events are italicized.

Notes: "NA" means not applicable. "Unknown" means not included in source document. Off-label use of a prescription drug or device refers to the ability of licensed health care providers to prescribe or use the drug for indications, conditions, patients, dosages or routes of administration not yet evaluated and approved by the FDA as part of a new drug approval application. Drug Shortage designation is based on either a specific discussion of those issues in the article or a third-party source, such as the FDA, the American Health-System Pharmacists or professional article. Specific sources for the reports of adverse events are listed below:

[a] Information is still emerging about this incident and the information listed here is incomplete.

[b] CDC, "Multistate fungal meningitis outbreak investigation," http://www.cdc.gov/HAI/outbreaks/meningitis.html and see http://www.fda.gov/Drugs/DrugSafety/ucm270296.htm. See footnote 36 for discussion of drug shortage.

[c] S. Huang, et al., "Notes from the field: Multistate outbreak of post procedural fungal endophthalmitis associated with a single compounding pharmacy," Morbidity and Mortality Weekly Report (MMWR), vol. 61, no. 17 (March-April 20 1 2), pp. 31 0-3 1 1. See also, FDA http://www.fda.gov/Safety/MedWatch/SafetyInformation/SafetyAlertsforHumanMedicalProducts/ucm296383.htm.

[d] R. A. Goldberg et al., "An Outbreak of Streptococcus Endophthalmitis After Intravitreal Injection of Bevacizumab," American Journal of Ophthalmology, (February, 20 1 2), pp. 204-208; A. B. Frost and M. A. Kainer, "Safe Preparation and Administration of Intravitreal Bevacizumab Injections," New England Journal of Medicine, vol. 365, no. 23 (December 201 1), 2238.

[e] Department of Veterans Affairs, Office of Inspector General, "Healthcare Inspection Oversight Review of Ophthalmology, Adverse Drug Events, VA Greater Los Angeles Healthcare System, Los Angeles, California." Report No. 1 2-0 1515- 15 1, (April 12, 20 1 2), http://www.va.gov/oig/pubs/VAOIG- 1 2-015 15-15 1.pdf.

[f] FDA: Safety: Meds IV Pharmacy, IV Compounded Products Recall; and N. Gupta et al., "Investigation of an outbreak of Serratia marcescens Bloodstream infections in patients receiving total parenteral nutrition – Alabama,1 ",201 Authors affiliated

with CDC and Alabama Dept. of Health, Paper presented at conference IDSA, October, 201 1, https://idsa.confex.com/idsa/201 1 /webprogram/Paper31248. html; and C. A. Thompson, "Bacteremia outbreak tied to improper filtration by compounding pharmacy," American Journal of Health System Pharmacy, vol. 68, no. 22, (201 1), pp. 21 10-1 1, http://www.ashp.org/menu/News/PharmacyNews/.

[g] B. Vitello, "Lutheran General to pay $8.25 million in baby's death," Daily Herald, April 5, 2012. http://www.dailyherald.com/article/20120405/news/704059806/.

[h] N. J. McKeown et al., "Deaths from intravenous colchicine resulting from a compounding pharmacy error – Oregon and Washington," Morbidity and Mortality Weekly Report, vol. 56, no. 40, (October 12, 2007), pp. 1050-1052, http://www.cdc.gov/mmwr/preview/mmwrhtml/mm5640a3.htm.

[i] L.A. Maragakis et al., "Sphingomonas paucimobilis Bloodstream infections associated with contaminated intravenous fentanyl," Emerging Infectious Disease, vol. 15, no. 1 (2009), pp. 12- 1 8, and FDA, http://www.fda.gov/downloads/Drugs/GuidanceComplianceRegulatoryInformation/PharmacyCompounding/UCM338614.pdf.

[j] M. S. McCoy, "Compounded Colistimethate as Possible Cause of Fatal Acute Respiratory Distress Syndrome" New England Journal of Medicine, vol. 357, no. 22 (November 29, 2007), pp. 231 0-23 1 1.

[k] L.A. Maragakis et al., "Sphingomonas paucimobilis Bloodstream infections associated with contaminated intravenous fentanyl," Emerging Infectious Disease, vol. 15, no. 1 (2009), pp. 12- 1 8, and FDA, http://www.fda.gov/downloads/Drugs/GuidanceComplianceRegulatoryInformation/PharmacyCompounding/UCM338614.pdf.

[l] Institute for Safe Medication Practices. Medication Safety Alert. "Failed check system for chemotherapy leads to pharmacist's no contest plea for involuntary manslaughter," April 23, 2009. http://www.ismp.org/newsletters/acutecare/articles/20090423.asp. Accessed January 9, 2013.

[m] M. Grissinger, "A Fatal Zinc Overdose in a Neonate. Confusion of Micrograms with Milligrams," Pharmacy and Therapeutics, vol. 36, no. 7, (July 2011), pp. 393-394, 409.

[n] J. F. Perz et al. "Pseudomonas putida Septicemia in a Special Care Nursery Due to Contaminated Flush Solutions Prepared in a Hospital Pharmacy," Journal of Clinical Microbiology, vol. 43, no. 10, (October 2005), pp. 5316-5318.

[o] Maryland State Board of Pharmacy. "Order for Summary Suspension." In the matter of Central Admixture Pharmacy Services, Inc. http://www.dhmh.maryland.gov/pharmacy/docs/FormalOrders/C/C.A.P.S%2011-15-05.pdf.

[p] R. Sunenshine et al., "An Outbreak of Postoperative Gram-Negative Bacterial Endophthalmitis Associated with Contaminated Trypan Blue Ophthalmic Solution," Clinical Infectious Diseases, vol. 48, no. 11, (April 2009), pp. 1580-1583.

[q] R. H. Sunenshine et al., "A Multi-state Outbreak of Serratia marcescens Bloodstream Infection Associated with Contaminated Intravenous Magnesium Sulfate from a

Compounding Pharmacy." Clinical Infectious Disease, vol. 45, (2007), pp. 527-533.

[r] M. R. Held et al., "Life-threatening sepsis caused by Burkholderia cepacia from contaminated intravenous flush solutions prepared by a compounding pharmacy in another state," Pediatrics, vol. 118, no. 1(July 1, 2006), pp. e212 -e215.

[s] U.S. Centers for Disease Control and Prevention, "Pseudomonas Bloodstream Infections Associated with a Heparin/Saline Flush—Missouri, New York, Texas, and Michigan, 2004–2005," Morbidity and Mortality Weekly Report, vol. 54, no. 11 (March 2005), pp. 269-272; and U.S. Centers for Disease Control and Prevention, "Update: Delayed Onset Pseudomonas fluorescens Bloodstream Infections After Exposure to Contaminated Heparin Flush—Michigan and South Dakota, 2005– 2006," Morbidity and Mortality Weekly Report, vol. 55, no. 35 (September 2006), pp. 961-963.

[t] Patel, P.R. et al., "Hepatitis C Virus Infections from a Contaminated Radiopharmaceutical Used in Myocardial Perfusion Studies," Journal of the American Medical Association, (October 6, 2006), vol. 296, pp. 2005-2011.

[u] CDC, "Exophilia Infection from Contaminated Injectable Steroids Prepared by a Compounding Pharmacy –United States," July-November 2002. MMWR, 51(49) (December 13, 2002), pp.1109-1112.

[v] R. Civen et al., "Outbreak of Serratia marcescens infections following injection of betamethasone compounded at a community pharmacy," Clinical Infectious Disease, vol. 43, no. 7 (August 22, 2006), pp. 831-837.

[w] D. Selenic et al., "Enterobacter cloacae bloodstream infections in pediatric patients traced to a hospital pharmacy," American Journal of Health System Pharmacies, vol.14, no. 60 (July 14, 2003), pp.1440-1446.

End Notes

[1] For more information on the events relating to tracking the fungal meningitis outbreak, see Beth Bell, Director, Director, National Center for Emerging and Zoonotic Diseases, Centers for Disease Control and Prevention (CDC), Department of Health and Human Services (HHS), "Testimony Before the Health, Education, Labor, and Pensions Committee, U.S. Senate: The CDC and Public Health Response to the 2012 Fungal Meningitis and Other Infections Outbreak," pp. 2-6, http://www.help.senate.gov/imo/media/doc/Bell.pdf.

[2] This form of fungal meningitis is non-contagious; the more common form of meningitis is bacterial and is infectious. See http://www.cdc.gov/meningitis/fungal.html.

[3] Centers for Disease Control and Prevention (CDC), Multistate Fungal Meningitis Outbreak Investigation—Current Case Count, accessed June 3, 2012, http://www.cdc.gov/hai/outbreaks/meningitis.html. This case count is updated monthly on the CDC website.

[4] Centers for Disease Control and Prevention, Multistate Fungal Meningitis Outbreak Investigation, accessed May 6, 2012, http://www.cdc.gov/HAI/outbreaks/currentsituation/; see also, http://www.cdc.gov/hai/outbreaks/meningitismap.html.

[5] Statement of Margaret Hamburg before the Senate Committee on Health, Education, Labor, and Pensions "Pharmacy Compounding: Implications of the 2012 Meningitis Outbreak," November 15, 2012, http://www.fda.gov/NewsEvents/ Testimony/ucm327667.htm; A. Goodnough, "Sterility Found Lacking at Drug Site in Outbreak," New York Times, October 23, 2012, http://www.nytimes.com/2012/10/24/health/sterility-found-lacking-at-drug-site-in-meningitisoutbreak.html?ref=health.

[6] The Food and Drug Administration (FDA) defines a serious adverse event as any undesirable experience associated with the use of a medical product in a patient. For more information, see FDA "What is a Serious Adverse Event?" http://www.fda.gov/safety/medwatch/ howtoreport/ucm053087.htm.

[7] See FDA, "Pharmacy Compounding" http://www.fda.gov/drugs/Guidance Compliance RegulatoryInformation/ PharmacyCompounding/default.htm.

[8] In 2003 another hearing was held: "Examining State and Federal Oversight to Ensure the Safety and Quality of Drug Compounding," hearing of the Senate Committee on Health, Education, Labor, and Pensions, 108th Congress, 1st Session, October 22, 2003.

[9] Office of the Inspector General, Memorandum Report: High-Risk Compounded Sterile Preparations and Outsourcing by Hospitals that Use Them, Department of Health and Human Services, OEI-01-13-00150, Washington, DC, April 1, 2013; K. Fiore, "Drug Shortages Spark Use of Compounders," (October 18, 2012), http://www.medpagetoday.com/ MeetingCoverage/ASA/35406.

[10] An adverse event involving the same type of contaminated compounded drug and fungal infection was reported as recently as May 24, 2013, see FDA, "Main Street Family Pharmacy in Tennessee: FDA Alerts Health Care Providers of Adverse Reactions Associated with Steroid Injections," http://www.fda.gov/Safety/MedWatch/ Safety Information/ SafetyAlertsforHumanMedicalProducts/ucm353953.htm.

[11] M.R. Cohen, "Meningitis cases spotlight broken system," Philly.com, October 17, 2012, http://www.philly.com/ philly/health/Meningitis-cases-spotlight-broken-system.html.

[12] J. Aleccia, "Fungal Meningitis Outbreak Tied to Steroid Shots, Isn't the First, Reports Show," October 18, 2012, http://vitals.nbcnews.com/_news/2012/10/18/14517177-fungal-meningitis-outbreak-tied-to-steroid-shots-isnt-the-firstreports-show?lite.

[13] Ibid., p. 5.

[14] An expanded overview of events related to the 2012 fungal meningitis outbreak can be found in CRS Report R42837, Selected Resources on Federal Oversight of Compounding Pharmacies, by Judith M. Glassgold, Susan Thaul, and Janet Kinzer.

[15] Beth Bell, Director, National Center for Emerging and Zoonotic Diseases, Centers for Disease Control and Prevention, HHS, "Testimony Before the Health, Education, Labor, and Pensions Committee, U.S. Senate: The CDC and Public Health Response to the 2012 Fungal Meningitis and Other Infections Outbreak," p. 6, http://www.help.senate.gov/imo/ media/doc/Bell.pdf.

[16] See CDC "Related Drug Recalls" http://www.cdc.gov/hai/outbreaks/ currentsituation/ archive.html, accessed May 6, 2012.

[17] For information on Congressional concerns regarding drug compounding that led to Section 503A, see U.S. Congress, Senate Committee on Labor and Human Resources, Food and Drug Modernization and Accountability Act of 1997, S. 830, 105th Cong., 1st sess., July 1, 1997, S.Rept. 105-43, pp. 67-69. For information on recent concerns with some references to the history of federal oversight, see "Pharmaceutical Compounding: Proposed Legislative Solution," hearing of the Committee on Health, Education, Labor, and Pensions, U.S. Senate, May 9, 2013; "A Continuing Investigation into the Fungal Meningitis Outbreak and

Whether It Could Have Been Prevented?", hearing of the Subcommittee on Oversight and Investigations, Committee on Energy and Commerce, U.S. House of Representatives, April 26, 2013; "Pharmacy Compounding: Implications of the 2012 Meningitis Outbreak," hearing of the Committee on Health, Education, Labor, and Pensions, U.S. Senate, November 15, 2012; "The Fungal Meningitis Outbreak: Could It Have Been Prevented?", hearing of the Subcommittee on Oversight and Investigations, Committee on Energy and Commerce, U.S. House of Representatives, November 14, 2012 "Examining State and Federal Oversight to Ensure the Safety and Quality of Drug Compounding."

[18] See US Pharmacopeial Convention-NF, General Chapter <797> Pharmaceutical Compounding – Sterile Preparations and USP-NF <795> Non-Sterile Compounding.

[19] See FDA, "Results" of "Report: Limited FDA Survey of Compounded Drug Products," http://www.fda.gov/Drugs/ GuidanceComplianceRegulatoryInformation/PharmacyCompounding/ucm204237.htm; "Stabilityhttp://www.fda.gov/Drugs/GuidanceComplianceRegulatoryInformation/Pharmacy Compounding/ucm204237.htm.

[20] Ibid., and FDA, "Results of Report: Limited FDA Survey of Compounded Drug Products," http://www.fda.gov/ Drugs/GuidanceComplianceRegulatoryInformation/PharmacyCompounding/ucm155725.ht m.

[21] See National Council of State Legislators, "State Regulation of Compounding Pharmacies," http://www.ncsl.org/ issues-research/health/regulating-compounding-pharmacies.aspx; Statement and response to questions, Janet Woodcock, FDA at a hearing of the Senate Committee on Health, Education, Labor and Pensions, "Pharmaceutical Compounding: Proposed Legislative Solution," May 9, 2013.

[22] Pew Charitable Trusts, American Society of Health-System Pharmacists, and American Hospital Association, "Pharmacy Compounding Summit: Summary of a Stakeholder Meeting," February 6, 2013, Washington, DC, p.3.

[23] A report from Rep. Markey's office details safety issues brought to state boards and transmitted to that office, see http://markey.house.gov/sites/markey.house.gov /files/ documents/Compounding%20Pharmacies%20- %20Compounding%20Risk%20FINAL_0.pdf.

[24] See Missouri Board of Pharmacy annual reports 2006-2011, http://pr.mo.gov/pharmacists-annual-reports.asp.

[25] T. Mullarkey, "Pharmacy Compounding of High-Risk Products and Patient Safety," American Journal of Health-System Pharmacists, vol. 66 (Suppl5), (September 1, 2009), p. S9.

[26] See discussion of limited state resources in the public meeting: "Framework for Pharmacy Compounding: State and Federal Roles," December 19, 2012, starting on p. 22, http://www.fda.gov/downloads/NewsEvents/MeetingsConferencesWorkshops/UCM3357 91. pdf.

[27] E. Dexheimer, "As Pharmacies Face Scrutiny, State Oversight Drops," Austin Statesman, November 3, 2012, accessed May 20, 2013. See also, National Association of Boards of Pharmacy, "Texas Board Surveys Pharmacies About Compounding Practices, Will Seek Legislative Support for Additional Inspectors," http://www.nabp.net/news/ texas-board-surveys-pharmacies-about-compounding-practices-will-seek-legislative-support-for-additional-inspectors, accessed May 20, 2013.

[28] Statement and response to questions, Janet Woodcock, FDA at a hearing of the Senate Committee on Health, Education, Labor and Pensions, "Pharmaceutical Compounding: Proposed Legislative Solution," May 9, 2013.

[29] U.S. General Accounting Office, Prescription Drugs: State and Federal Oversight of Drug Compounding by Pharmacies, 04-195T, September 23, 2003, http://www.gao.gov/products/GAO-04-195T.

[30] Information on these concerns can be found on FDA webpages of adverse events, warning letters, manufacturer recall notices, and in professional journals. See section: "Articles from Legal, Professional, and Scientific Journals" in CRS Report R42837, Selected Resources on Federal Oversight of Compounding Pharmacies, by Judith M. Glassgold, Susan Thaul, and Janet Kinzer; and FDA, "Results" of "Report: Limited FDA Survey of Compounded Drug Products," http://www.fda.gov/Drugs/GuidanceComplianceRegulatory Information/ PharmacyCompounding/ucm155725.htm.

[31] For a selected group of resources see CRS Report R42837, Selected Resources on Federal Oversight of Compounding Pharmacies, by Judith M. Glassgold, Susan Thaul, and Janet Kinzer; also, FDA "Pharmacy Compounding," http://www.fda.gov/Drugs/GuidanceComplianceRegulatoryInformation/PharmacyCompounding/ default.htm; and FDA, "Introduction: 2006 Limited FDA Survey of Compounded Drug Products," http://www.fda.gov/Drugs/GuidanceComplianceRegulatoryInformation/PharmacyCompounding/ucm204237.htm.

[32] Off-label use of a prescription drug or device refers to the ability of licensed health care providers to prescribe or use the drug for indications, conditions, patients, dosages or routes of administration not yet evaluated and approved by the FDA as part of a new drug approval application.

[33] Sterile compounding differs from non-sterile compounding. When compounding exclusively with sterile ingredients, sterility must be maintained in all phases of production; when compounding with non-sterile ingredients, sterility must be achieved for the finished product. These processes require special equipment, facilities, and personnel training. See T. Mullarkey, "Pharmacy Compounding of High-Risk Products and Patient Safety," American Journal of Health-System Pharmacists, vol. 66 (Suppl5), (September 1, 2009), p. s5; see USP-NF, "General Chapter <797> Pharmaceutical Compounding – Sterile Preparations," http://www.usp.org/store/products-services/usp-compounding.

[34] E. S. Kastango, American Society of Health-System Pharmacists, "The ASHP Discussion Guide for Compounding Sterile Preparations," http://www.ashp.org/s_ashp/docs/files/HACC_797guide.pdf.

[35] Some reports included concerns with products, but no adverse events. See for instance, M.P. Goldman, "Sodium Tetradecyl Sulfate for Sclerotherapy Treatment of Veins: Is Compounded Pharmacy Solution Safe?" American Society for Dermatologic Surgery, vol. 30, pp. 1454-1456; K. Hundley, "Lincare Pharmacy Runs Afoul of Missouri Regulators," St. Petersburg Times, April 18, 2003; S. Sellars and W.H. Utian, "Pharmacy Compounding Primer for Physicians: Prescriber Beware, " Drugs, vol. 72, no. 16, pp. 2043-2050.

[36] In early 2012, Hospira was listed on the FDA shortages website as discontinuing methylprednisolone: http://www.fda.gov/drugs/drugsafety/drugshortages/ucm050794.htm. Another site reports a shortage of methylprednisolone in May 2012, http://eraycollins.blogspot.com/2012/05/shortage-of-injectable.html; and K. Kindy, L.H. Sun, and A. Crites, "Compounding pharmacies have been linked to deaths, illnesses, and safety failures for years," Washington Post, February 7, 2013, http://articles.washingtonpost.com/2013-02-07/national/36970682_1_medicationsfor-individual-patients-massachusetts-pharmacy-meningitis-outbreak.

[37] See Testimony of Margaret Hamburg at a hearing of the Subcommittee on Oversight and Investigations, Committee on Energy and Commerce, U.S. House of Representatives, "A

Continuing Investigation into the Fungal Meningitis Outbreak and Whether It Could Have Been Prevented?", April 26, 2013.

[38] FDA, 2013 Inspections, http://www.fda.gov/AboutFDA/Centers Offices/ Office ofGlobalRegulatoryOperationsandPolicy/ORA/ORAElectronicReadingRoom/ucm340853.htm, accessed May 6, 2012 and http://www.fda.gov/Safety/Recalls/default.htm, accessed May 6, 2012.

[39] Ibid.

[40] See FDA, http://www.fda.gov/Safety/MedWatch/SafetyInformation/SafetyAlertsfor Human MedicalProducts/ ucm353953.htm.

[41] This list of recalled CD is current as of May 31, 2013. Additional notices can be found at http://www.fda.gov/Safety/ MedWatch/default.htm.

[42] See FDA, http://www.fda.gov/Safety/Recalls/ucm354450.htm.

[43] See FDA, http://www.fda.gov/Safety/MedWatch/SafetyInformation/SafetyAlertsfor Human MedicalProducts/ ucm353953.htm.

[44] See FDA, http://www.fda.gov/Safety/Recalls/ucm354182.htm?source=govdelivery.

[45] See FDA http://www.fda.gov/Safety/ Medatch/Safety Information/SafetyAlertsforHuman MedicalProducts/ ucm352939.htm.

[46] See FDA http://www.fda.gov/Safety/Recalls/ucm351841.htm.

[47] See http://www.fda.gov/Safety/Recalls/ucm349040.htm.

[48] See http://www.fda.gov/Safety/Recalls/ucm348723.htm.

[49] See FDA Recalls: http://www.fda.gov/Safety/Recalls/ucm348095.htm.

[50] See FDA http://www.fda.gov/Safety/MedWatch/SafetyInformation/Safety Alerts for HumanMedicalProducts/ ucm352949.htm?source=govdelivery.

[51] See FDA Recalls: http://www.fda.gov/Safety/Recalls/ucm348094.htm.

[52] See FDA Recalls: http://www.fda.gov/Safety/Recalls/ucm347559.htm.

[53] C. Conaboy and K. Lazar, "State Halts Drug Production at Woburn Pharmacy," Boston Globe, March 24, 2013, http://bostonglobe.com/lifestyle/health-wellness/2013/03/25/ woburn-compounding-pharmacy-issues-recall-sterile-products/j7QDTvv5WIHO1FU8W6mNGP/story.html.

[54] See FDA http://www.fda.gov/Drugs/DrugSafety/DrugRecalls/.

[55] See FDA "Recall – Firm Press Release", http://www.fda.gov/Safety/Recalls/ ucm34478 6. htm?source=govdelivery.

[56] See FDA Recalls http://www.fda.gov/Safety/Recalls/ucm344377.htm.

[57] FDA, "Medprep Consulting Inc. Announces Voluntary Nationwide Recall of all Lots of all Compounded Products Due to Potential Mold Contamination," March 17, 2013, http://www.fda.gov/Safety/Recalls/ucm344787.htm.

[58] See FDA Recall: http://www.fda.gov/Safety/Recalls/ucm344189.htm.

[59] "Thompson v. Western States," 535 U.S. 357 at 360-361.

[60] Ibid.

[61] Ibid., p. 361. Cost may be a factor in certain circumstances, see D. J. DeNoon, reviewed by L.J. Martin, "FDA: Pharmacies Can Still Make Preterm Birth Drug," http://www. webmd.com/baby/news/20110330/fda-generic-makenaok; and "FDA Statement on Makena" http://www.fda.gov/NewsEvents/Newsroom/PressAnnouncements/ ucm 2790 98.htm.

[62] Statement and response to questions, Janet Woodcock, FDA at a hearing of the Senate Committee on Health, Education, Labor and Pensions, "Pharmaceutical Compounding: Proposed Legislative Solution," May 9, 2013.

[63] Comments of Margaret Hamburg, Commissioner of Food and Drugs, FDA, transcript of public meeting "Framework for Pharmacy Compounding: State and Federal Roles," December 19, 2012.

[64] Testimony of Steven Galson, FDA, at a hearing of the Senate Committee on Health, Education, Labor, and Pensions, 108th Congress, 1st Session, October 22, 2003, "Examining State and Federal Oversight to Ensure the Safety and Quality of Drug Compounding."

[65] Since close to 4 billion prescriptions are filled annually in the United States, this percentage would yield a range of 40-200 million CDs annually.

[66] P. M. Barrett, "America's Shadow Pharmacies," Bloomberg Businessweek, November 14, 2012; and Denise Grady, Sabrina Tavernise, and Andrew Pollack, "In a Drug Linked to a Deadly Meningitis Outbreak, a Question of Oversight," New York Times, October 4, 2012, http://www.nytimes.com/2012/10/05/health/news-analysis-a-question-of-oversighton-compounding-pharmacies.html. Another estimate of 30-50 million annually is from the FDA, see Testimony of Steven Galson, FDA, at a hearing of the Senate Committee on Health, Education, Labor, and Pensions, 108th Congress, 1st Session, October 22, 2003, "Examining State and Federal Oversight to Ensure the Safety and Quality of Drug Compounding."

[67] States license health care professionals. The scope of permitted activities of pharmacy professionals is largely determined by state law. For an example of a job description for a compounding professional, see http://www.wedgewoodpharmacy.com/jobs/pharmacy-technician-general-compounding.html, accessed April 1, 2013.

[68] National Council of State Legislators, "State Regulation of Compounding Pharmacies," http://www.ncsl.org/issuesresearch/health/regulating-compounding-pharmacies.aspx.
Telephone conversation between the author and Joe Cabaleiro, Executive Director, Pharmacy Compounding Accreditation Board, January 4, 2013; and, see American Pharmacists Association, "Frequently Asked Questions about Pharmaceutical Compounding," http://www.pharmacist.com/frequently-asked-questions-about-pharmaceutical-compounding, accessed May 20, 2013.

[69] Pew Charitable Trusts, American Society of Health-System Pharmacists, and American Hospital Association, "Pharmacy Compounding Summit: Summary of a Stakeholder Meeting," February 6, 2013, Washington DC.

[70] Steven Galson, FDA, at a hearing of the Senate Committee on Health, Education, Labor, and Pensions, 108th Congress, 1st Session, October 22, 2003, "Examining State and Federal Oversight to Ensure the Safety and Quality of Drug Compounding." The FDA provided limited information on this study, so its reliability cannot be assessed.

[71] See J. Woodcock interview with an industry newsletter, Pharmalot: http://www.lawofcompoundingmedications.com/ 2013/04/during-pharmalot-interview-fda.html.

[72] See http://www.pharmacist.com/compounding-just-the-facts.

[73] See the International Academy of Compounding Pharmacies website, http://www.iacprx.org.

[74] Telephone conversation between the author and Joe Cabaleiro, Executive Director, Pharmacy Compounding Accreditation Board, January 4, 2013.

[75] Products provided by compounding pharmacies can be found on websites generated by standard searches of the web with keywords such as "compounding pharmacies." Further, the website of the Pharmacy Compounding Accreditation Board, a private non-profit organization that accredits compounding pharmacies has a list of accredited compounding pharmacies, http://www.pcab.org/. A list of products provided by compounded pharmacies can be found on the websites of accredited members, see for instance, CarePro

Compounding. http://www.careprohs.com/pharmacies/ compounding/ or A & O pharmacy, http://www.aopharmacy.com/compounding.html.

[76] Statement of K. Thompson, American Society of Health-System Pharmacists, hearing of Committee on Health, Education, Labor, and Pensions, U.S. Senate, November 12, 2012, http://www.help.senate.gov/imo/media/doc/ Thompson7.pdf.

[77] FDA Actions, http://www.fda.gov/Drugs/GuidanceComplianceRegulatory Information/ PharmacyCompounding/ #compliance See list of resources in CRS Report R42837, Selected Resources on Federal Oversight of Compounding Pharmacies, by Judith M. Glassgold, Susan Thaul, and Janet Kinzer for examples of medical and scientific journals and FDA resources.

[78] For more information, see the following compounding pharmacies' websites: http://www.pccarx.com/join-pcca/; http://www.moorespharmacy.com/testimonials.htm; and http://www.hotzehwc.com/en-US/Treatment-Programs/ FAQ.aspx.

[79] For example, see the following compounding pharmacy website: http://www.myvillagegreen.com/compoundingpharmacy/.

[80] For example, see the following compounding pharmacy http://www.hotzehwc.com/en-US/Treatment-Programs/ Adrenal-Fatigue.aspx.

[81] In some instances the FDA has issued warning letters to compounding pharmacies regarding the claims of these products. For example, see FDA, "FDA Issues Warning Letters for Drugs Promoted in Fat Elimination Procedure," press release, April 7, 2010, http://www.fda.gov/NewsEvents/Newsroom/PressAnnouncements/2010/ucm207453.htm.

[82] "FDA Warns Marketers of Unapproved 'Chelation' Drugs, http://www.fda.gov/ ForConsumers/ConsumerUpdates/ ucm229358.htm; FDA Warning Letter CIN-10-94106-12, Libido Edge Labs, LLC, 06/10/2010; R. Sood et al., "Counseling Postmenopausal Women About Bio-Identical Hormones: Discussion Point 10: Adrenal Fatigue Does Not Mean Adrenal Insufficiency," Journal of the Board of Family Medicine, vol. 24, no. 2, (2011), pp. 202-210;

[83] See for instance, objections by compounding pharmacies to FDA regulation, including Medical Ctr. Pharm., 536 F.3d and Franck's Lab, 816 F. Supp. 2d.

[84] The term "non-traditional" compounding is found in a number of sources: Comments of Margaret Hamburg, Commissioner of Food and Drugs, FDA, transcript of public meeting "Framework for Pharmacy Compounding: State and Federal Roles," December 19, 2012); Office of the Inspector General, Memorandum Report: High-Risk Compounded Sterile Preparations and Outsourcing by Hospitals that Use Them, Department of Health and Human Services, OEI-01-13-00150, Washington, DC, April 1, 2013. Another term used for this activity is "compounding manufacturing" (Source: S. 959 introduced by Senator Harkin and passed out of Committee by the Senate Committee on Health, Education, Labor and Pensions circulated in the 113th Congress).

[85] Parenteral nutrition is IV administered nutrition, which bypasses the digestive tract.

[86] See PharMedium, "Compounding Services," http://www.pharmedium.com/ compounding/ index.html, accessed May 20, 2013.

[87] Pew Charitable Trusts, American Society of Health-System Pharmacists, and American Hospital Association, "Pharmacy Compounding Summit: Summary of a Stakeholder Meeting," February 6, 2013, Washington DC, p. 7.

[88] See FDA http://www.fda.gov/downloads/Drugs/DrugSafety/ FungalMeningitis/ UCM3254 66.pdf, accessed May 20, 2013.

[89] Unless otherwise noted this section is based on CRS Report R43038, Federal Authority to Regulate the Compounding of Human Drugs, by Andrew Nolan. For more information, see

CRS Report R43038, Federal Authority to Regulate the Compounding of Human Drugs, by Andrew Nolan, and CRS Report R40503, FDA's Authority to Regulate Drug Compounding: A Legal Analysis, by Jennifer Staman.

[90] Ibid., see the above reports for a discussion of Section 503A.

[91] See generally Franck's Lab, 816 F. Supp. 2d at 1235-1239 (discussing the cases that have examined the scope of the FDA's authority with respect to compounding).

[92] See e.g., Wedgewood Village Pharmacy, 421 F.3d at 272-73.

[93] See CPG §460.200 (May 29, 2002); see also CPG §608.400 (July 14, 2003).

[94] W. States Med. Ctr., 535 U.S. at 361.

[95] R.R. Abood, Pharmacy Practice and the Law, 6th ed. Sudbury, MA: Jones and Bartlett (2011).

[96] This report is not meant to be a comprehensive survey of state law regulations on pharmacy compounding. For more information on the topic, the National Conference of State Legislatures provides summaries of existing state laws and new initiatives. See "State Regulation of Compounding Pharmacies," updated April 13, 2013, http://www.ncsl.org/issues-research/health/regulating-compounding-pharmacies.aspx.

[97] Ibid.

[98] See National Association of Boards of Pharmacies, http://www.nabp.net/news/tagged/compounding.

[99] Ibid.

[100] See, e.g., Fla. Admin. Code Ann. 64B16-27.700(1)(c).

[101] See, e.g., 49 Pa. Code § 27.18(p)(2); W. Va. Code St. Rules, tit. 15, § 19.4.

[102] See, e.g., Okla. Admin. Code §§ 535:15-10-3, 535:15-10-9(d); Colorado State Board of Pharmacy Rule 3.02.10.

[103] See for instance, California Business and Professional Code Section 4127 regarding standards for compounding injectable sterile products, http://www.leginfo.ca.gov/cgi-bin/displaycode?section=bpc&group=04001-05000&file= 4127-4127.8, accessed May 21, 2013.

[104] See New Jersey 13:39-4.18(a) et seq. Procedures for Centralized Prescription Handling, http://www.njconsumeraffairs.gov/adoption/pharmado_100509.htm.

[105] See H.2. "The Pharmacy Act and Drug Control Act with Related Statutes", Commonwealth of Virginia, (July 1, 2012), http://www.dhp.virginia.gov/Pharmacy/pharmacy _laws_ regs.htm.

[106] W. States Med. Ctr., 535 U.S. at 361 (noting that as a "traditional component of the practice of pharmacy, compounding is taught as a part of the standard curriculum at most pharmacy schools.")

[107] The U.S. Pharmacopeial Convention (USP) is a scientific nonprofit organization that sets standards for the identity, strength, quality, and purity of medicines, food ingredients, and dietary supplements manufactured and distributed worldwide. USP's drug standards are referenced in FFDCA. The Pharmacy Compounding Accreditation Board (PBAB) sets standards for compounding, http://www.pcab.org/.

[108] See National Conference of State Legislatures, "State Regulation of Compounding Pharmacies, Updated April 16, 2013.

[109] See USP-NF, "General Chapter <797> Pharmaceutical Compounding – Sterile Preparations," (Date), Appendix A.

[110] Ibid., p. 9.

[111] Pew Charitable Trusts, American Society of Health-System Pharmacists, and American Hospital Association, "Pharmacy Compounding Summit: Summary of a Stakeholder Meeting," February 6, 2013, Washington DC, p. 8.

[112] Ibid.

[113] See also FDA "Facts About Current Good Manufacturing Practices" http://www.fda.gov/drugs/ developmentapprovalprocess/manufacturing/ucm169105.htm

[114] J. Lee, "Investors Buying Compounders," ModernHealthcare.com, January 19, 2013, http://www.modernhealthcare.com/article/20130119/MAGAZINE/301199973; F. Gebhart, "Flush with victory, compounding pharmacists see demand soar," Drug Topics, vol. 144, no. 2 (January 17, 2000), pp. 28-31; and testimony by Steven Galson, FDA, before the Senate Committee on Health, Education, Labor, and Pensions, October 23, 2003, http://www.fda.gov/NewsEvents/Testimony/ucm115010.htm.

[115] J. Lee, "Investors Buying Compounders," ModernHealthcare.com, January 19, 2013, http://www.modernhealthcare.com/article/20130119/MAGAZINE/301199973.

[116] E.S. Kastango, "Outsourced Medications: How Can You Know They Are Safe?" Clinical IQ, 2013, http://pharmacyonesource.com/images/simplifi797/Outsourcing-Meds.pdf.

[117] T. Mullarkey, "Considerations in Pharmacy Compounding and the Treatment of Spasticity, Introduction," American Journal of Health-System Pharmacies, vol. 66 (Suppl5), s2-3; V. Yancey et al., "Perceptions of Pharmaceutical Care Among Pharmacists Offering Compounding Services," Journal of the American Pharmaceutical Association, vol. 48, pp. 508-514 (2008); R. Jones, "Custom Cures," Wayne State Alumni Magazine, spring 2010, pp. 10-11, http://mydigimag.rrd.com/publication/index.php?i=37104&m=&l= &14&pre=&ver=swf&p=10; and Professional Compounding Centers of America, "Compounding and Pharmacists," http://www.pccarx.com/pharmacists/.

[118] Statement and response to questions, Janet Woodcock, FDA at a hearing of the Senate Committee on Health, Education, Labor and Pensions, "Pharmaceutical Compounding: Proposed Legislative Solution," May 9, 2013.

[119] See FDA website "2013 Pharmacy Inspections," http://www.fda.gov/Drugs /GuidanceComplianceRegulatoryInformation/PharmacyCompounding/ucm339771.htm, accessed May 30, 2013.

[120] K. Kindy, L.H. Sun, and A. Crites, "Compounding pharmacies have been linked to deaths, illnesses, and safety failures for years," Washington Post, February 7, 2013, http://articles.washingtonpost.com/2013-02-07/national/ 36970682_1_medications-for-individual-patients-massachusetts-pharmacy-meningitis-outbreak; C. Lomax, "IV Outsourcing: Doing More with Less," White Paper, Pharmacy Purchasing and Products, http://www.pppmag.com/ white_papers/.

[121] A central fill pharmacy is defined as a pharmacy which is permitted by the state in which it is located to prepare prescriptions on behalf of a retail pharmacy (pursuant to a valid prescription) to be distributed by the retail pharmacy to the patient if the two pharmacies have a contractual agreement. See for instance, 21 CFR 1300.01 "Definitions."

[122] "Outsourcing pharmacy" refers to the transmitting of a prescription order from a primary pharmacy to a secondary "outsourcing" pharmacy that prepares the prescription. See for instance: Maryland Office of the Secretary of State, http://www.dsd. state.md.us/comar/SubtitleSearch.aspx?search=10.34.04.

[123] See New Jersey 13:39-4.18(a) et seq. Procedures for Centralized Prescription Handling, http://www.njconsumeraffairs.gov/adoption/pharmado_100509.htm.

[124] FDA, "Medprep Consulting Inc. Announces Voluntary Nationwide Recall of all Lots of all Compounded Products Due To Potential Mold Contamination," March 17, 2013, http://www.fda.gov/Safety/Recalls/ucm344787.htm.

[125] Telephone conversation between author and Joe Cabaleiro, Executive Director, Pharmacy Compounding Accreditation Board, January 4, 2013. Recent amendments to the FFDCA require more extensive tests and labeling for prescription drugs for children. For more

information about prescription drugs for children see CRS Report RL33986, FDA's Authority to Ensure That Drugs Prescribed to Children Are Safe and Effective, by Susan Thaul, and CRS Report R42680, The Food and Drug Administration Safety and Innovation Act (FDASIA, P.L. 112-144), coordinated by Susan Thaul.

[126] Such drugs include epidurals for pain management during childbirth or chronic pain conditions, and chemotherapy.

[127] Pew Charitable Trusts, American Society of Health-System Pharmacists, and American Hospital Association, "Pharmacy Compounding Summit: Summary of a Stakeholder Meeting," February 6, 2013, Washington DC, p. 5.

[128] Ibid., p. 4; K. Douglass and E.S. Kastango, "Consolidation of Pharmacy Compounding Services: An Alternative to Outsourcing," International Journal of Pharmaceutical Compounding, vol. 5, no. 2 (March/April 2001), pp. 140-144, http://www.clinicaliq.com/content/consolidation.pdf.

[129] Ibid. See also Pew Charitable Trusts, American Society of Health-System Pharmacists, and American Hospital Association, "Pharmacy Compounding Summit: Summary of a Stakeholder Meeting," February 6, 2013, Washington, DC.

[130] Pew Charitable Trusts, American Society of Health-System Pharmacists, and American Hospital Association, "Pharmacy Compounding Summit: Summary of a Stakeholder Meeting," February 6, 2013, Washington, DC, p. 4.

[131] Products for an individual patient include anti-infectives, pain management therapies, chemotherapy drugs, replacement fluids and electrolytes, and ophthalmic preparations. See Pharmacy Compounding Summit: Summary of a Stakeholder Meeting, Pew Charitable Trusts, American Society of Health-System Pharmacists, and American Hospital Association, February 6, 2013, Washington DC, p. 4.

[132] Pew Charitable Trusts, American Society of Health-System Pharmacists, and American Hospital Association, "Pharmacy Compounding Summit: Summary of a Stakeholder Meeting," February 6, 2013, Washington, DC, p. 4.

[133] Ibid., p. 5, see text related to Prattville Baptist Hospital.

[134] See, C. Lomax, "IV Outsourcing: Doing More with Less," White Paper, Pharmacy Purchasing and Products, http://www.pppmag.com/white_papers/; Pew Charitable Trusts, American Society of Health-System Pharmacists, and American Hospital Association, "Pharmacy Compounding Summit: Summary of a Stakeholder Meeting," February 6, 2013, Washington, DC, p. 5.

[135] Office of the Inspector General, Memorandum Report: High-Risk Compounded Sterile Preparations and Outsourcing by Hospitals that Use Them, Department of Health and Human Services, OEI-01-13-00150, Washington, DC, April 1, 2013, p. 4.

[136] Ibid., p. 6.

[137] E.S. Kastango, 2013; and C.Y. Johnson, "Compounding Pharmacies Fill Important Medical Niche," Boston Globe, November 3, 2012, http://www.bostonglobe.com/metro/2012/11/02/compounding-pharmacies-filled-niche-for-major-hospitals/47MsPtBMEkT67TQmfNXF8O/story.html; K. Fiore, "Drug Shortages Spark Use of Compounders," (October 18, 2012), http://www.medpagetoday.com/Meeting Coverage/ASA/35406; and T. Meyer, "Overseeing Outsourced Compounding During Shortages," Pharmacy Purchasing and Products, June 2012, http://www.pppmag.com /article/1141/June_2012/Overseeing_Outsourced_Compounding_during_Shortages/#.T9k83KBsIlQ.blogger; K. Thomas, "Lapses at Big Drug Factories Add to Shortages and Danger," New York Times, October 17, 2012, http://www.nytimes.com/2012/10/18/

business/drug-makers-stalled-in-a-cycle-of-quality-lapses-and-shortages.html?pagewanted=all.

[138] K. Thomas, "Lapses at Big Drug Factories Add to Shortages and Danger," New York Times, October 17, 2012, http://www.nytimes.com/2012/10/18/business/drug-makers-stalled-in-a-cycle-of-quality-lapses-and-shortages.html? pagewanted=all.

[139] See Wedgewood Pharmacy, "Drug Shortages and Alerts," http://www.wedgewoodrx.com/healthcare-professionals/ current-drug-shortages-and-alerts.html, and http:// www.wedgewoodpharmacy.com/news/press-room/wedgewoodpharmacy-compounds-gentamicin-as-sulfate-40mg-ml-injection-solution-during-manufacturer-.html, accessed April 1, 2013; Preckshot Professional Pharmacy http://www.preckshotpharmacy.com/rss2html.php?XMLFILE=http:// www.pharmdjd.com/u/rss/meds_s.xml&TEMPLATE=unavailable_medications.html,accessed April 5, 2013; Universal Arts Pharmacy http://www.uaprx.com/, accessed April 5, 2013.

[140] J. Lee, "Investors Buying Compounders," ModernHealthcare.com, January 19, 2013, http://www.modernhealthcare.com/article/20130119/MAGAZINE/301199973; K. Fiore, "Drug Shortages Spark Use of Compounders," October 18, 2012, http://www.medpagetoday.com/MeetingCoverage/ASA/35406; and T. Meyer, "Overseeing Outsourced Compounding During Shortages," Pharmacy Purchasing and Products, June 2012, http://www.pppmag.com/article/1141/June_2012/Overseeing_Outsourced_ Compounding_during_Shortages/ #.T9k83KBsIlQ.blogger. Sections 1001-1008 of the Food Drug Safety and Administration Act (P.L. 112-144) included provisions to ease shortages, see FDA website http://www.fda.gov/RegulatoryInformation/Legislation/ FederalFoodDrugandCosmeticActFDCAct/SignificantAmendmentstotheFDCAct/FDASIA/ucm313121.htm.

[141] K. Thomas, "Drug Shortages Persist in U.S., Harming Care," New York Times, November 16, 2012, http://www.nytimes.com/2012/11/17/business/drug-shortages-are-becoming-persistent-in-us.html?pagewanted=all& _r=0&pagewanted=print; K. Fiore, "Drug Shortages Spark Use of Compounders," October 18, 2012, http://www.medpagetoday.com/MeetingCoverage/ASA/35406; and T. Meyer, "Overseeing Outsourced Compounding during Shortages," Pharmacy Purchasing and Products, June 2012, http://www.pppmag.com /article/1141/June_2012/ Overseeing_Outsourced_Compounding_during_Shortages/#.T9k83KBsIlQ.blogger.

[142] Office of the Inspector General, Memorandum Report: High-Risk Compounded Sterile Preparations and Outsourcing by Hospitals that Use Them, Department of Health and Human Services, OEI-01-13-00150, Washington, DC, April 1, 2013.

[143] See comments of Margaret Hamburg, Commissioner of Food and Drugs, FDA, transcript of public meeting "Framework for Pharmacy Compounding: State and Federal Roles," December 19, 2012.

[144] See FDA Recalls: K. Thomas, "Lapses at Big Drug Factories Add to Shortages and Danger," New York Times, October 17, 2012, http://www.nytimes.com/2012/10/18/business/drug-makers-stalled-in-a-cycle-of-quality-lapses-andshortages.html?pagewanted=all.

[145] See FDA Recalls: http://www.fda.gov/Drugs/DrugSafety/DrugRecalls/.

[146] J. Woodcock and M. Wosinska, "Economic and Technological Drivers of Generic Sterile Injectable Drug Shortages," Clinical Pharmacology and Therapeutics," vol. 93, no. 2, (February 2013), pp.170-176.

[147] Ibid.

[148] E. Palmer, "Compounder Recall May Make Drug Shortages More Severe," FiercePharmaManufacturing, October 31, 2012, http://www.fiercepharmamanufac turing.com/story/compounder-recall-may-make-drug-shortages-moresevere/2012-10-31.

[149] K. Thomas, "Lapses at Big Drug Factories Add to Shortages and Danger," New York Times, October 17, 2012, http://www.nytimes.com/2012/10/18/business/drug-makers-stalled-in-a-cycle-of-quality-lapses-and-shortages.html? pagewanted=all.

[150] See FDA Drug Recalls, http://www.fda.gov/Drugs/DrugSafety/DrugRecalls/.

[151] Compare FDA, "Drug Shortage Index," March 11, 2013, http://www.fda.gov/ drugs/drugsafety/drugshortages/ ucm050792.htm, with list of drugs recalled by Med Prep, March 17, 2013, http://www.fda.gov/Safety/Recalls/ ucm344229.htm.

[152] E. Palmer, "Compounder Recall May Make Drug Shortages More Severe," FiercePharmaManufacturing, October 31, 2012, http://www.fiercepharmamanufac turing.com/story/compounder-recall-may-make-drug-shortages-moresevere/2012-10-31; Y. Johnson, "Compounding Pharmacies Fill Important Medical Niche," Boston Globe, November 3, 2012, http://www.bostonglobe.com/metro/2012/11/02/compounding-pharmacies-filled-niche-for-major-hospitals/ 47MsPtBMEkT67TQmfNXF8O/story.html.

[153] K. Cubert, "Compounding Pharmacies in the US: Doctor's orders: Drug Shortages and Demand from the Aging Population Will Benefit Stores," IBIS World Industry Report OD5706, May 2012, pp. 10-11; see also, FDA "How Widespread is the Marketing of Compounded "BHRT" drugs?"; http://www.fda.gov/Drugs/ GuidanceCompliance RegulatoryInformation/PharmacyCompounding/ucm183088.htm; and a compounding pharmacy site, Precision Compounding Pharmacy: http://www.precisioncom pounding pharmacy.com/?q=bhrt.

[154] The FDA has issued warnings about the evidence of the usefulness or uniqueness of CDs for these indications. FDA, see "Bio-Identicals: Sorting Myths from Facts," http:/ /www.fda. gov/ForConsumers/ConsumerUpdates/ ucm049311.htm.

[155] V. Yancey et al., "Perceptions of Pharmaceutical Care Among Pharmacists Offering Compounding Services," Journal of the American Pharmacists Association, vol. 48, no. 4 (Jul/Aug 2008), pp. 508-514; and R. Jones, "Custom Cures," Wayne State Alumni Magazine, spring 2010, pp. 10-11, http://mydigimag.rrd.com/publication/index.php?i= 37104&m=&l=&14&pre=&ver=swf&p=10.

[156] See for instance. Chain Drug Review, "2012 Retail Forecast: Chain Drug Eyes Broader Role," http://www.chaindrugreview.com/inside-this-issue/news/01-02-2012/2012-retail-forecast-chain-drug-eyes-broaderrole; Council on Credentialing in Pharmacy, "Scope of Contemporary Pharmacy Practice: Roles, Responsibilities, and Functions of Pharmacists and Pharmacy Technicians, Journal of the American Pharmacy Association, vol. 50, no. 2 (March-April, 2010), e35-e69.

[157] P.M. Barrett, "America's shadow pharmacies," Business Week, http://www.businessweek. com/articles/2012-11-14/ americas-shadow-pharmacies.

[158] For instance, see Kelley Ross https://www.krrph.com/about-us/history.aspx, accessed March 31, 2013.

[159] Ibid., and R. Dresser & J. Frader, "Off-label prescribing: A Call for Heightened Professional and Governmental Oversight," Journal of Law and Medical Ethics, vol. 37, no. 3, pp. 476-486.

[160] R. Lowes, "Compounding Pharmacy Crackdown Continues with Avastin Recall," http://www.medscape.com/ viewarticle/781039 accessed May 20, 2013; J. B. Staal et al., "Injection therapy for subacute and chronic low back pain: An updated Cochrane Review,"

Spine, vol. 34, no. 1 (January 2009), pp. 49-59. Evidence differs on whether these off-label treatments are effective.

[161] Ibid.

[162] See CDC, Multistate Fungal Meningitis Outbreak Investigation - Current Situation, http://www.cdc.gov/HAI/ outbreaks/currentsituation/.

[163] See T. Mullarkey, "Pharmacy Compounding of High-Risk Products and Patient Safety," American Journal of Health-System Pharmacists, vol. 66 (Suppl5), (September 1, 2009), p. s5; see USP-NF, "General Chapter <797> Pharmaceutical Compounding – Sterile Preparations," http://www.usp.org/store/products-services/usp-compounding.

[164] Office of the Inspector General, Memorandum Report: High-Risk Compounded Sterile Preparations and Outsourcing by Hospitals that Use Them, Department of Health and Human Services, OEI-01-13-00150, Washington, DC, April 1, 2013; "FDA Concept Paper: Drug Products That Present Demonstrable Difficulties for Compounding Because of Reasons of Safety and Effectiveness," updated 04/20/2009, http://www.fda.gov/ RegulatoryInformation/ Legislation/FederalFoodDrugandCosmeticActFDCAct/SignificantAmendmentstotheFDCAct/FDAMA/ ucm100205.htm; comments of Margaret Hamburg, Commissioner of Food and Drugs, FDA, transcript of public meeting "Framework for Pharmacy Compounding: State and Federal Roles," December 19, 2012, pp. 10; and see USPNF, "General Chapter <797> Pharmaceutical Compounding – Sterile Preparations," http://www.usp.org/store/products-services/usp-compounding.

[165] Statement and response to questions, Janet Woodcock, FDA at a hearing of the Senate Committee on Health, Education, Labor and Pensions, "Pharmaceutical Compounding: Proposed Legislative Solution," May 9, 2013, http://www.help.senate.gov/hearings/hearing/ ?id=f9b68c5e-5056-a032-52b6-4e632afd726a.

[166] For more information, see hearing of the Senate Committee on Health, Education, Labor and Pensions, "Pharmaceutical Compounding: Proposed Legislative Solution," May 9, 2013, http://www.help.senate.gov/hearings/hearing/?id=f9b68c5e-5056-a032-52b6-4e632afd726a.

[167] See statements and response to questions of Panel 2 at "Pharmaceutical Compounding: Proposed Legislative Solution," a hearing of the Senate Committee on Health, Education, Labor and Pensions, May 9, 2013, http://www.help.senate.gov/hearings/hearing/?id= f9b68c5e-5056-a032-52b6-4e632afd726a.

[168] Adverse events are reported to poison control centers, FDA, CDC, or state public health authorities. Adverse event reporting is required for commercially-manufactured drugs (21 U.S.C. §355-1), non-prescription drugs (21 U.S.C. §379aa), and dietary supplements (21 U.S.C. §379aa-1); for more information see, CRS Report R41983, How FDA Approves Drugs and Regulates Their Safety and Effectiveness, by Susan Thaul and CRS Report R43062, Regulation of Dietary Supplements, by Amalia K. Corby-Edwards. Also see Guidance for Industry http://www.fda.gov/downloads/ Drugs/GuidanceCompliance RegulatoryInformation/Guidances/UCM299138.pdf; FDA Adverse Event Reporting System http://www.fda.gov/drugs/guidancecomplianceregulatoryinformation/surveillance/adversedrugeffects/ default.htm.

[169] A few, but not all, states require some form of reporting of adverse incidents from CDs, see National Council of State Legislators, "State Regulation of Compounding Pharmacies," http://www.ncsl.org/issues-research/health/ regulating-compounding-pharmacies.aspx; see for instance, Massachusetts http://www.mass.gov/eohhs/docs/dph/ quality/boards/ necc/121101-pharmacy-board-draft-emergency-regs.pdf, and Texas http://law.onecle.com/ texas/ occupations/562.153.00.html.

[170] Statement and response to questions, Janet Woodcock, FDA at a hearing of the Senate Committee on Health, Education, Labor and Pensions, "Pharmaceutical Compounding: Proposed Legislative Solution," May 9, 2013.

[171] See http://www.fda.gov/Safety/MedWatch/default.htm.

[172] Statement and response to questions, Janet Woodcock, FDA at a hearing of the Senate Committee on Health, Education, Labor and Pensions, "Pharmaceutical Compounding: Proposed Legislative Solution," May 9, 2013. H.R. 6584and H.R. 6638 were introduced in the 112th Congress. In the 113th Congress, S. 959 was introduced by Senator Harkin. An Executive Committee hearing was held and the legislation in the 113th Congress by Representative Markey; this bill includes provisions that provide for patient information on whether a drug is compounded in labeling.

[173] Statement and response to questions, Janet Woodcock, FDA at a hearing of the Senate Committee on Health, Education, Labor and Pensions, "Pharmaceutical Compounding: Proposed Legislative Solution," May 9, 2013.

[174] See for instance "Pharmacy Compounding: Facts and Information," specifically "When Are Compounded Drugs Necessary," and "Disclosure" http://www.ppsinc.org/phcom/03risk.htm; and M. R. Cohen, "New legislation would help users identify source of a compounded drug," Philly.com, http://www.philly.com/philly/blogs/healthcare/New-legislation-would-help-users-identify-source-of-a-compounded-drug.html#D0rsmdaRGFqMCMWT.99.

[175] T. L. Beauchamp and J. F. Childress, Principles of Biomedical Ethics, 9th ed. (New York: Oxford University, 2009).

[176] See for instance "Pharmacy Compounding: Facts and Information," specifically "When Are Compounded Drugs Necessary," and "Disclosure" http://www.ppsinc.org/phcom/03risk.htm; and M. R. Cohen, "New Legislation Would Help Users Identify Source of a Compounded Drug," Philly.com, http://www.philly.com/philly/blogs/healthcare/New-legislation-would-help-users-identify-source-of-a-compounded-drug.html#D0rsmdaRGFq MCMWT.99.

[177] See transcripts of: "A Continuing Investigation into the Fungal Meningitis Outbreak and Whether It Could Have Been Prevented?", hearing of the Subcommittee on Oversight and Investigations, Committee on Energy and Commerce, U.S. House of Representatives, April 26, 2013; "Pharmacy Compounding: Implications of the 2012 Meningitis Outbreak," hearing of the Committee on Health, Education, Labor, and Pensions, U.S. Senate, November 15, 2012; "The Fungal Meningitis Outbreak: Could It Have Been Prevented?" hearing of the Subcommittee on Oversight and Investigations, Committee on Energy and Commerce, U.S. House of Representatives, November 14, 2012; "Examining State and Federal Oversight to Ensure the Safety and Quality of Drug Compounding." hearing of the Senate Committee on Health, Education, Labor, and Pensions, 108th Congress, 1st Session, October 22, 2003.

[178] For instance, see Testimony of Margaret Hamburg, Commissioner of Food and Drugs, before the Committee on Health, Education, Labor, and Pensions, U.S. Senate, November 15, 2012, http://www.fda.gov/NewsEvents/Testimony/ ucm327667.htm; Statement of Margaret Hamburg before the Subcommittee on Oversight and Investigations, Committee on Energy and Commerce, U.S. House of Representatives, November 14, 2012, http://www.fda.gov/NewsEvents/Testimony/ucm327664.htm; and, Steven Galson, FDA, at a hearing of the Senate Committee on Health, Education, Labor, and Pensions, 108th Congress, 1st Session, October 22, 2003, "Examining State and Federal Oversight to Ensure the Safety and Quality of Drug Compounding."

[179] Ibid.

[180] See S. 959 introduced by Senator Harkin and passed out of the Senate Committee for Health, Education, Labor, and Pensions.

[181] See H.R. 6584 introduced by Representative Markey and H.R. 6638 introduced by Representative DeLauro in the 112th Congress, and H.R. 2186 introduced by Representative Markey in the 113th Congress.

[182] See S. 959 introduced by Senator Harkin and passed out of the Senate Committee for Health, Education, Labor, and Pensions.

[183] U.S. Congress, House Committee on Energy and Commerce, Subcommittee on Oversight and Investigations, Majority Memorandum RE: Hearing on "The Fungal Meningitis Outbreak: Could It Have Been Prevented?", November 12, 2012 and "A Continuing Investigation into the Fungal Meningitis Outbreak and Whether It Could Have Been Prevented?", hearing of the Subcommittee on Oversight and Investigations, Committee on Energy and Commerce, U.S. House of Representatives, April 26, 2013.

[184] U.S. Congress, House Committee on Energy and Commerce, Subcommittee on Oversight and Investigations, Majority Memorandum RE: Hearing on "The Fungal Meningitis Outbreak: Could It Have Been Prevented?", prepared by Subcommittee on Oversight and Investigations Staff, 112th Cong., 2nd sess., November 12, 2012, pp. 25, http://energycommerce.house.gov/sites/republicans.energycommerce.house.gov/files/Hearings/OI/20121114/HMTG112-HHRG-IF02-20121114-SD001.pdf.

[185] Ibid., pp. 6-23.

[186] Testimony from David Miller, International Academy of Compounding Pharmacists, Committee on Health, Education, Labor, and Pensions, "Pharmacy Compounding Implications of the 2012 Meningitis Outbreak," November 15, 2012, http://www.help.senate.gov/imo/media/doc/Miller8.pdf.

[187] See Panel II statements and response to questions, "Pharmaceutical Compounding: Proposed Legislative Solution," a hearing of the Committee on Health, Education, Labor, and Pensions, May 9, 2013; Press Release, PharMedium, March 26, 2013, http://www.lawofcompoundingmedications.com/2013/03/pharmedium-supports-new-fdacategory.html, accessed May 3, 2013.

[188] Pew Charitable Trusts, American Society of Health-System Pharmacists, and American Hospital Association, "Pharmacy Compounding Summit: Summary of a Stakeholder Meeting," February 6, 2013, Washington DC, p. 14.

In: Drug Compounding
Editor: Martti Bram

ISBN: 978-1-63117-360-8

Chapter 2

FEDERAL AUTHORITY TO REGULATE THE COMPOUNDING OF HUMAN DRUGS*

Andrew Nolan

SUMMARY

In light of the 2012 fungal meningitis outbreak, believed to have been caused by a contaminated compounded steroid injection, the regulation of human drug compounding has received significant attention. Drug compounding in its traditional form is the process of combining, mixing, or altering ingredients in order to create a medication for a particular patient. However, as illustrated by the entity that created the steroid medication linked with the meningitis outbreak, concerns have been raised about compounding pharmacies producing drugs on a larger scale. While drug compounding has historically been the focus of state governments through their regulation of pharmacies, questions have arisen regarding the extent the federal government can regulate the practice of compounding through the Food, Drug, and Cosmetic Act (FDCA).

Federal authority over compounding largely stems from the FDCA, enacted in 1938, and its subsequent amendments, including the Food and Drug Administration Modernization Act (FDAMA) of 1997, which added compounding specific provisions to the FDCA in Section 503A. A First

* This is an edited, reformatted and augmented version of a Congressional Research Service publication, CRS Report for Congress R43038, prepared for Members and Committees of Congress, from www.crs.gov, dated April 12, 2013.

Amendment challenge to Section 503A's advertising provisions and a resulting Supreme Court decision has created a split amongst the federal courts regarding whether Section 503A has any legal effect. The legal uncertainty regarding Section 503A, coupled with Section 503A's basis in the FDCA's "new drug," "adulteration," and "misbranding" provisions lends to an examination of the scope of federal authority under the base statute. Courts appear to agree that the federal government can regulate compounding activity that is akin to manufacturing, and courts have afforded deference to the FDA's interpretation of when a compounder is acting like a manufacturer. However, uncertainty remains regarding the possible limits to the FDA's power to regulate traditional compounding activities. This report will examine the FDA's regulation of drug compounding and will discuss relevant legal authorities. The report will conclude by discussing potential limits to the FDA's authority to regulate human drug compounding.

BACKGROUND

Drug compounding traditionally refers to the process in which a pharmacist combines, mixes, or alters various ingredients to create a medication that is "tailored to the needs" of an individual patient.[1] Compounding is generally used to prepare medications that are not commercially available, such as a drug in a lower dosage for a child, or a drug without a dye or a preservative in response to a patient allergy.[2]

Recent events have refocused attentions on compounding and the federal role in regulating drug compounding. In the fall of 2012, the Food and Drug Administration (FDA) and the Centers for Disease Control and Prevention (CDC) identified the presence of bacterial and/or fungal contamination in steroid injections from a New England compounding pharmacy.[3] The contamination has been linked with a multistate fungal meningitis outbreak that resulted in over 50 deaths.[4]

As a consequence, questions have arisen regarding the safety of compounded drugs and the role of federal and state governments in regulating compounded drugs and compounding pharmacies. Congressional hearings held by the Energy and Commerce Committee of the U.S. House of Representatives and the Health, Education, Labor, and Pensions Committee of the U.S. Senate probed the current policy and legal questions prompted by the meningitis outbreak.[5] One of the issues raised at these hearings was the extent of federal authority over compounding.[6] During these hearings, the Commissioner of the FDA noted the need for clarification and strengthening of the FDA's authority to "prevent" contaminations caused by compounding from occurring in the future,[7] while other representatives of professional associations contended that existing FDA authorities were adequate to have prevented the 2012 outbreak.[8] Thus, in the wake of the 2012 meningitis outbreak, a central issue that this report explores is the nature and scope of federal authority to regulate entities that compound drugs for humans.

FEDERAL REGULATION OF COMPOUNDED DRUGS

Compounding Before the 1938 Food, Drug, and Cosmetic Act

At the inception of the modern federal drug law, compounding was practiced extensively and widely regulated by the states.[9] On June 30, 1906, Congress enacted the Pure Food and Drug Act,[10] the first significant drug legislation that attempted to address the problems of drug safety and effectiveness. However, the Pure Food and Drug Act, which was passed with the purpose to "secure the purity of food and drugs and to inform purchasers of what they are buying,"[11] did not mandate a federal premarket approval or notification system for new drugs, let alone attempt to substantively regulate drug compounding. Instead, the 1906 act was concerned with false labeling of food and drugs, and as long as a drug compounder made no false or misleading claims with regard to the ingredients in a product, the compounder's actions would not run afoul of the Pure Food and Drug Act.[12] The advent of modern federal regulation of drugs arrived 22 years later when Congress enacted the Food, Drug, and Cosmetic Act (FDCA).[13]

The 1938 Food, Drug, and Cosmetic Act

The Food, Drug, and Cosmetic Act of 1938 established a complex and comprehensive scheme for regulating drugs that are distributed in interstate commerce.[14] While the 1938 act on its face is silent with respect to compounding,[15] three provisions are particularly relevant to the subject. First, the act defines a "new drug" as "[a]ny drug ... not generally recognized ... as safe ... for use under the conditions prescribed, recommended, or suggested in the labeling thereof."[16] The statute forbids introducing any "new drug" into interstate commerce without FDA approval.[17] Under current law, to obtain FDA approval, the sponsor must submit an extensive application to the FDA containing data that demonstrate that the new drug is both safe and effective for its intended uses in humans and that it will be manufactured such that the drug will preserve its identity, strength, quality, and purity.[18]

In addition to the act's "new drug" provisions, the current version of the FDCA has "adulteration" provisions that deem a drug to be "adulterated" if, among other things, the drug and the methods used in its creation do not conform with "current good manufacturing practices" that ensure the product's safety and quality.[19] The FDA has promulgated regulations that describe current good manufacturing practices.[20] Those regulations include, for example, requirements that the equipment used in the manufacturing of drugs be cleaned or sterilized at certain times[21] and that records related to manufacturing practices be maintained for at least a year after the expiration date of a batch of drugs.[22]

Third, the 1938 act contains provisions that discuss when a drug is "misbranded."[23] In relevant part, a drug can be "misbranded" if the drug's labeling[24] fails to bear "adequate directions for use."[25] FDA regulations generally define "adequate directions for use" as directions under which a layperson can use a drug "safely and for which it is intended."[26] Federal regulations further note several examples of when a direction may be "inadequate," such as the omission of "all" purposes for which the drug is intended[27] or the incorrect specification of the time of administration of a drug.[28]

Section 301 of the FDCA prohibits an individual from introducing or delivering into interstate commerce (1) a "new drug" without prior FDA approval,[29] (2) an "adulterated" drug,[30] or (3) a "misbranded" drug.[31] That same section also prohibits the "adulteration" or "misbranding" of a drug in interstate commerce,[32] the "receipt in interstate commerce of" an adulterated or misbranded drug, and the manufacturing of any adulterated or misbranded drugs.[33] The FDCA authorizes the United States to seek injunctive relief in federal court to restrain any violations of Section 301,[34] and the law subjects individuals who have violated the FDCA's prohibitions to civil fines and criminal penalties.[35] Furthermore, Section 304 of the FDCA allows the United States to proceed against and seize mislabeled or adulterated drugs.[36]

The breadth of the FDCA's "new drug," "adulteration," and "misbranding" provisions, on their face, have the potential to touch on local, traditional compounding efforts.[37] However, for nearly 50 years following the passage of the FDCA, the FDA did not use the FDCA's "new drug," "adulteration," or "misbranding" provisions as a means to regulate the practice of compounding.[38] Instead, the "FDA generally left regulation of compounding to the States," and "[p]harmacists continued to provide patients with compounded drugs without applying for FDA approval of those drugs."[39] The rationale for the FDA's initial approach toward drug compounding was that it is widely recognized that compounded drugs could not meet the FDCA's "new drug" requirements.[40] As the Supreme Court has noted, subjecting compounding pharmacies to the statute's approval requirements "would as a practical matter, eliminate the practice of compounding, and thereby eliminate availability of compounded drugs for those patients who have no alternative treatment."[41] This is because FDA approval requires "proof of the safety and effectiveness of a new drug ... [as] established by rigorous, scientifically valid clinical studies," a process that is extremely time consuming and costly.[42] As the Court observed, it is neither medically practicable nor "economically feasible" to subject compounded medications to the type of testing required by the FDCA for a new drug approval;[43] "requiring such testing would force pharmacists to stop providing compounding drugs."[44]

Kefauver-Harris Drug Amendments of 1962

The Kefauver-Harris Drug Amendments of 1962 (Drug Amendments), enacted in the wake of the thalidomide crisis of the early 1960s, constituted the first mentioning of compounding in federal drug law.[45] In relevant part, the Drug Amendments required manufacturers and others to register their establishments and strengthened the ability of the FDA to conduct on-site inspections.[46] The Drug Amendments, however, exempted "pharmacies ... which do not ... compound, or process drugs for sale other than in the regular course of their business of dispensing or selling drugs at retail" from registration requirements[47] and from enhanced inspections of a pharmacy's books and records.[48] Case law interpreting the Drug Amendments of 1962, however, has held that federal authorities have the right to enter establishments involved in the production of drugs to inspect equipment, materials, containers, and labeling used in the production process.[49]

Food and Drug Administration Modernization Act of 1997 and Compounding

In 1997, Congress amended the FDCA through the Food and Drug Administration Modernization Act (FDAMA).[50] The amendment contained provisions on drug compounding that resulted, in part, from a growing concern that an "increasing number of establishments with retail pharmacy licenses [were] engaged in manufacturing and distributing unapproved new drugs for human use in a manner that was clearly outside the bounds of traditional pharmacy practice."[51]

Put another way, the FDA was concerned that "some pharmacists were manufacturing and selling drugs under the guise of compounding," as a way of avoiding the FDCA's "new drug," "adulteration," and "misbranding" provisions.[52] Accordingly, the intent of the FDAMA's compounding provisions was "to clarify the application of the [FDCA] to professional practice of pharmacists' compounding of drug products."[53]

To do so, the FDAMA explicitly deems that three provisions of the FDCA are inapplicable to drug compounding that complies with various requirements.[54]

The three provisions are the FDCA's provisions on (1) the sale of a "new drug," (2) adulteration and the need to adhere to "good manufacturing practices," and (3) misbranding and the need to provide "adequate directions for use" on a drug.[55] With respect to requirements for compounding, the law requires that compounding be done by a licensed pharmacist or physician in response to a valid prescription for an identified individual patient, or, if prepared before the receipt of such a prescription, the drug be made in only "limited quantities" and in response to a history of the licensed pharmacist's or physician's receipt of valid prescription orders for that drug product within an established relationship between the pharmacist, the patient, and the prescriber.[56]

Additionally, the law requires that the compounded drug be made from approved ingredients that meet certain standards, and the compounded drug may not appear on an FDA list of drug products that have been withdrawn or removed from the market because they were found to be unsafe or ineffective.[57] The FDAMA also prohibits the compounding of drugs in "inordinate amounts" such that the drugs are "essentially copies of a commercially available drug product."[58] The law also allows the FDA to identify certain drug products that present "demonstrable difficulties" for compounding in terms of safety or effectiveness, prohibiting the compounding of such articles.[59] In states that have not entered into an agreement with the FDA addressing the distribution of "inordinate amounts" of compounded drugs in interstate commerce, the pharmacy, pharmacist, or physician compounding the drug may not distribute compounded drugs out of state in quantities exceeding 5% of that entity's total prescription orders.[60]

FDAMA and Federal Authority After *Thompson v. Western States Medical Center*

The FDAMA also included a ban on advertising by compounders.[61] However, in 2003, the Supreme Court in *Thompson v. Western States Medical Center* invalidated the FDAMA's advertising provisions on First Amendment grounds.[62] Generally, if a part of a law is held to be unconstitutional, the unconstitutional provision is "severable" or "dropped" from what remains of a law unless it is "evident that the Legislature would not have enacted" the remaining provisions independently of the unconstitutional provision.[63] In the wake of *Western States,* a split has emerged amongst the federal circuit court of appeals about whether the remaining provisions of the FDAMA are "severable" from the advertising provision at issue in the *Western States* case.[64]

As a consequence, within the states within the Ninth Circuit,[65] the controlling precedent renders the remaining provisions of the FDAMA inoperable.[66] The opposite is true in the Fifth Circuit,[67] and the legal effect of the FDAMA is unresolved in the rest of the country.[68] The FDA noted in 2002, prior to the Fifth Circuit's decision, that in light of the Supreme Court decision, the FDAMA "is now invalid,"[69] and instead, the FDA "outlined the criteria"[70] it would use to assess "what types of compounding might be subject to enforcement under current law" (i.e., the FDCA)[71] in a 2002 Compliance Policy Guide (CPG).[72] In the wake of the Fifth Circuit's decision, the FDA has taken the position[73] that the agency "will apply the non-advertising provisions of section 503A to entities covered by this provision that are located within the jurisdiction of the Fifth Circuit ... as well as to the plaintiffs that brought the *Medical Center* case."[74]

The 2002 CPG was issued out of a "need for immediate guidance" for "the compounding industry on what factors the [FDA] will consider in exercising its enforcement discretion regarding pharmacy compounding."[75] The policy guidance generally notes while the FDA "will continue to defer to state authorities regarding less significant violations of the [FDCA] related to pharmacy compounding of human drugs,"[76] the agency will focus on "concerns normally associated with a drug manufacturer and result in significant violations of the new drug, adulteration, or misbranding provisions of the Act."[77] In determining whether to take an enforcement action against a compounding entity, the CPG notes nine non-exhaustive factors that will guide regulators.[78] The factors are summarized in *Table 1*.[79]

Table 1. Factors Guiding Whether the FDA Will Take Action Against a Compounder of Human Drugs

Is the compounding ... ?	If yes, is the FDA more likely to assert its regulatory authority?
... done in anticipation of receiving prescriptions?	No
... involving a drug that was withdrawn or removed from the market for safety reasons?[a]	Yes
... based from bulk active ingredients?	Yes (if not from a FDA-approved drug or without a FDA sanctioned New Drug Application)
... done without obtaining written assurance from the supplier that the drug substances were made in an FDA-registered facility?	Yes
... not in compliance with official compendia requirements?	Yes
... using commercial scale manufacturing or testing equipment?	Yes
... done for third parties who will resell the drugs?	Yes
... of drug products that are commercially available in the	Yes
marketplace or essentially copies of commercially available drugs?	
... failing to comply with applicable state law?	Yes

Source: Prepared by CRS.

Notes: Derived from FDA Compliance Policy Guide §460.200 (May 29, 2002).

[a] See 21 C.F.R. §216.24 (list of drug products withdrawn or removed from the market for reasons of safety or effectiveness).

In 2003, the FDA issued guidance with regard to veterinary compounding.[80] Similar to its 2002 guidance on human compounding, the FDA noted its concerns regarding compounding that is "clearly outside of the bounds of traditional pharmacy practice" and is "intended to circumvent [the FDCA's] drug approval process and provide for the mass marketing of products that have been produced with little to no quality control or manufacturing standards to ensure the purity, potency, and stability of the product."[81] The 2003 CPG announced that while the FDA will "generally" "defer to state authorities regarding the day-to-day regulation of compounding by veterinarians," federal authority will be asserted when the activities in question raise the "kinds of concerns normally associated with a drug manufacturer" and "result in significant violations of the new animal drug, adulteration, or misbranding provisions" of the act.[82] In determining whether to take an enforcement action against a compounding entity, the CPG on animal drug compounding notes 13 non-exhaustive factors that will guide regulators.[83] The factors largely mirror the concerns illustrated in the 2002 CPG for human drug compounding and include concerns common to both human and animal drug compounding.[84] For example, the FDA noted that the volume of drugs being compounded or whether the compounding used commercial scale manufacturing equipment would be used by federal officials when determining whether to take an enforcement action against an animal drug compounder.[85]

Both the 2002 and 2003 CPGs on drug compounding make clear that the FDA, as a matter of public policy, will focus its enforcement efforts on compounding efforts that are akin to "manufacturing" and will defer to state governments with respect to "traditional compounding."[86] As a matter of law, the FDA does not attempt, in the two CPGs, to limit its authority under the FDCA. Instead, the CPGs note that the FDCA does not "distinguish compounding from manufacturing"[87] and deem violations of the FDCA that do not relate to manufacturing to be a concern of "state authorities."[88]

LIMITS ON FEDERAL AUTHORITY TO REGULATE COMPOUNDED DRUGS

The legal uncertainty about the validity of the compounding provisions of the FDAMA, coupled with the FDA's renewed reliance on the FDCA's new drug, adulteration, and misbranding provisions as the source of the federal authority to regulate drug compounding, has prompted considerable discussion with respect to the extent of the FDA's authority under the 1938 act. Moreover, even if the FDAMA's compounding provisions still have legal effect, the provisions are based on blanket exemptions for certain compounding activity from the FDCA's new drug, adulteration, and misbranding requirements, all of which are based on the assumption that broad federal authority to regulate drug compounding exists.[89] With this backdrop, a debate has arisen regarding the limits of federal authority under the FDCA with respect to the regulation of drug compounding.

The FDA maintains the position that pharmacy-compounded drugs are "new drugs" or "new animal drugs" within the meaning of the FDCA,[90] and, therefore, the entire practice of compounding is "under FDA scrutiny."[91] According to the agency, as a "matter of discretion" the FDA has "historically declined" to take "enforcement action against pharmacies engaged in traditional drug compounding."[92] Pharmacists, in response, have disputed the reach of the FDA's authority, finding "cold comfort in the FDA's promised self-restraint."[93] Instead, those who oppose the FDA's theory of its authority to regulate compounding contend that the practice of compounding was widespread at the time of the 1938 act, and Congress would not have intended to expand the FDA's regulatory authority to make compounding activities covered by the act's new drug, adulteration, and misbranding provisions,[94] regulations that, if enforced literally, would functionally prohibit traditional compounding.[95]

Courts that have examined the issue have all agreed that the FDA has *some* authority to regulate compounding.[96] Specifically, case law appears to find that the FDCA does provide the federal government with the authority to prohibit pharmacists from manufacturing under the guise of compounding.[97] According to one recent court decision, "[t]o the extent that a pharmacist's bulk compounding activity moves beyond the bound of traditional compounding and begins to approximate the 'manufacturing' of unapproved drugs, there seems little question that this activity is squarely within the crosshairs of the FDCA."[98] Moreover, courts have interpreted the FDA's 2002 CPG as a reasonable means by which the FDA can gauge whether an entity is engaged in manufacturing.[99]

However, a question remains as to whether a so-called "maximalist" interpretation of the FDA's authority exists, such that any "traditional compounding" is "*per se* unlawful under the FDCA."[100] In favor of the maximalist interpretation of the FDA's authority over compounding is the plain language of the FDCA.[101] Specifically, the FDCA's "new drug" provisions broadly state that no person can "introduce or deliver for introduction into interstate commerce any new drug, unless an approval of an application filed" pursuant to the statute with the FDA has occurred with respect to the drug.[102] Moreover, Section 501 of the FDCA broadly deems a drug to be "adulterated" if it "is a drug and the" way it was manufactured, processed, packaged, or held does not conform with good manufacturing practices that ensure its quality and purity.[103] The FDCA's misbranding provisions are equally broad, in that the statute deems a drug to be "misbranded" if its labeling does not bear "adequate directions for use."[104] In none of the three aforementioned provisions does the FDCA's plain language exempt traditional compounding activity from the act's reach. As one court has noted, "[c]ompounded drugs are, after all, drugs,"[105] and therefore, the plain language of the statute would seem to indicate that compounding activities are within the purview of the FDA's authority under the act.[106] Moreover, the maximalist interpretation is supported by the argument that because exemptions exist under the FDCA's provisions for other types of drugs, such "investigational drugs,"[107] one can presume from Congress's refusal to create a general exemption for traditional compounding an implicit extension of federal authority over all forms of compounding.[108]

On the other hand, given the "ubiquity of pharmacy compounding at the time Congress passed the FDCA," it can be argued that it would be absurd for Congress to have taken the "unprecedented" action to implicitly regulate compounded drugs through the 1938 act.[109] This argument is buttressed by Supreme Court case law on statutory interpretation that generally holds that it should not be assumed that Congress "alter[s] the fundamental details of a regulatory scheme in vague terms or ancillary provisions."[110] Moreover, the legislative history of the FDCA appears to support the view that manufacturers were the intended target of the regulatory scheme imposed by the 1938 act.[111] For example, the then-President of the American Pharmaceutical Association testified before a Senate subcommittee in 1938 in support of the legislation that while the "regulations governing ... the practice of pharmacy are very strict ... the privileges of unlicensed persons operating outside of pharmacies are so extensive that the public enjoys little protection,"[112] evincing that Congress's central concern with the FDCA was manufacturing, not traditional pharmacy compounding. Legislative history can guide a court in assessing the correct interpretation of the scope of the FDA's authority under the act.[113]

The current limits of federal authority to regulate traditional drug compounding have been discussed by very few courts, and each court that has approached the issue did so from a unique factual setting that colored the eventual outcome of the case.[114] As a consequence, the precise limit to federal authority with respect to drug compounding remains uncertain, although Congress could arguably expand the scope of the FDCA to reach traditional compounding.[115] As a matter of policy, the FDA has generally declined to test the current limits of its authority to regulate compounding,[116] preferring to defer to state governments with respect to the regulation of "traditional compounding."[117] As a result, absent further congressional action, the limits of the FDA's authority to regulate all forms of compounding will likely continue to be unresolved.[118] With respect to enforcement efforts clearly within the FDA's broad discretion, such as combating compounding that is akin to large-scale manufacturing, courts will likely provide considerable deference to the FDA.[119]

End Notes

[1] See Thompson v. W. States Med. Ctr., 535 U.S. 357, 360-61 (2002).

[2] Id. at 361.

[3] Centers for Disease Control and Prevention, Multistate Fungal Meningitis Outbreak Investigation—Current Case Count, http://www.cdc.gov/hai/outbreaks/meningitis.html.

[4] Centers for Disease Control and Prevention, Multistate Fungal Meningitis Outbreak Investigation—Current Case Count, http://www.cdc.gov/hai/outbreaks/meningitis-map-large.html (noting that as of March 25, 2013, 730 cases of fungal infections had been linked to steroid injections, resulting in 51 deaths).

[5] See U.S. Congress, House Committee on Energy and Commerce, Subcommittee on Oversight and Investigations, The Fungal Meningitis Outbreak: Could It Have Been Prevented, 112th Cong., 2nd sess., November 14, 2012; see also U.S. Congress, Senate Committee on Health, Education, Labor, and Pensions, Pharmacy Compounding: Implications of the 2012 Meningitis Outbreak, 112th Cong., 2nd sess., November 15, 2012, http://www.help.senate.gov/hearings/hearing/?id=5f5def0d-5056-a032-5297-eab57634d 209.

[6] U.S. Congress, Senate Committee on Health, Education, Labor, and Pensions, Pharmacy Compounding: Implications of the 2012 Meningitis Outbreak, 112th Cong., 2nd sess., November 15, 2012, http://www.help.senate.gov/hearings/ hearing/?id=5f5def0d-5056-a032-5297-eab57634d209.

[7] See Margaret A. Hamburg, Testimony before U.S. Congress, Senate Health, Education, Labor and Pensions Committee, Pharmacy Compounding: Implications of the 2012 Meningitis Outbreak, 113th Cong., November 15, 2012, http://www.help.senate.gov/imo/media/doc/Hamburg3.pdf ("As described above, FDA's ability to take action against compounding that exceeds the bounds of traditional pharmacy compounding and poses risks to patients has been hampered by gaps and ambiguities in the law, which have led to legal challenges to FDA's authority to inspect pharmacies and take appropriate enforcement actions.")

[8] See, e.g., David Miller, International Academy of Compounding Pharmacists, Testimony before U.S. Congress, Senate Health, Education, Labor and Pensions Committee, Pharmacy Compounding: Implications of the 2012 Meningitis Outbreak, 113th Cong., November 15, 2012, http://www.help.senate.gov/imo/media/doc/Miller8.pdf the federal standpoint, the FDCA's existing inspection provision, section 704, allows FDA oversight when a pharmacy is not operating in conformity with governing state laws, or akin to a drug manufacturer.")

[9] See Joint Session of Am. Pharm. Ass'n, et al., 17 J. Am. Pharm. Ass'n 1000, 1010-13 (1938).

[10] P.L. 59-384, 34 Stat. 768 (1906).

[11] United States v. Antikamnia Chem. Co., 231 U.S. 654, 665 (1913)

[12] See James Harvey Young, The Toadstool Millionaires: A Social History of Patent Medicines in America Before Federal Regulation 9, 243-44 (Princeton Univ. Press. 1961).

[13] P.L.75-717, 52 Stat. 1057 (1938).

[14] See generally CRS Report R41983, How FDA Approves Drugs and Regulates Their Safety and Effectiveness, by Susan Thaul.

[15] United States v. Franck's Lab, Inc., 816 F. Supp. 2d 1209, 1254 n.7 (M.D. Fl. 2011) (noting that the FDCA is "silent on the topic" of compounding).

[16] 21 U.S.C. §321(p)(1). The "new drug" provision of the FDCA contains a "grandfather clause" that excludes drugs subject to regulation under a 1906 federal statute, if the labeling is appropriate. Id. The FDCA broadly defines the term "drug" to include "articles intended for use in the diagnosis, cure, mitigation, treatment or prevention of disease in man or other animals." 21 U.S.C. §321(g)(1)(B).

[17] 21 U.S.C. §§331(d), 355(a).

[18] 21 U.S.C. §§355(a)-(d). The FDCA has specific provisions that discuss the role of new animal drugs. Specifically, "new animal drugs" that have not been approved by the FDA are "unsafe" and "adulterated." See 21 U.S.C. §§351(a)(5) & 360b(a)(1)(A).

[19] 21 U.S.C. §351(a)(1)(B). The precursor to the modern language regarding "good manufacturing practices" in the 1938 Act were provisions that broadly deemed a drug to be "adulterated" if it had been "prepared, packed, or held under insanitary conditions ..." See P.L.75-717, §501(a)(2). The provision on "good manufacturing practices" resulted from the Kefauver-Harris Drug Amendments of 1962. See infra.

[20] See 21 C.F.R. parts 210, 211, 225, and 226.

[21] See 21 C.F.R. §211.67.

[22] See 21 C.F.R. §211.180.

[23] See 21 U.S.C. §352.

[24] Labeling is defined under the FFDCA to include "all labels and other written, printed, or graphic matters (1) upon any article or any of its containers or wrappers, or (2) accompanying such article." 21 U.S.C. §321(m). The Supreme Court, in Kordel v. United States, broadly interpreted the phrase "accompanying such article" to include materials that supplement or explain the product. 335 U.S. 345, 349 (1948).

[25] 21 U.S.C. §352(f)(1). The statute does allow the Secretary to promulgate regulations exempting a drug if providing "adequate directions for use" are not necessary for the "protection of public health." Id. 21 C.F.R. §201.122 exempts from the FDCA's "adequate directions for use" requirement drugs in bulk form intended for processing, repackaging or use in the "manufacture of another drug" if the bulk drug contains labeling that indicates its proper use. Id. However, the exemption only extends to a drug where an approved new drug application or new animal drug application or new animal drug index listing is affiliated with the production. See 21 C.F.R. 201.122(a)-(c).

[26] 21 C.F.R. §201.5.

[27] 21 C.F.R. §201.5(a).

[28] 21 C.F.R. §201.5(e). For example, a drug label could be inadequate if it incorrectly specifies that the drug should be taken with food. Id.

[29] 21 U.S.C. §301(d).

[30] 21 U.S.C. §301(a).

[31] 21 U.S.C. §301(a).

[32] 21 U.S.C. §301(b).

[33] 21 U.S.C. §301(c).

[34] 21 U.S.C. §332(a).

[35] See 21 U.S.C. §333.

[36] 21 U.S.C. §334(a).

[37] See Medical Ctr. Pharm. v. Mukasey, 536 F.3d 383, 395 (5th Cir. 2008) (noting the language of the FDCA's new drug definition to be "both plain and expansive"); United States v. Franck's Lab, Inc., 816 F. Supp. 2d 1209, 1237 (M.D. Fl. 2011) (noting that the FDCA's provision if "read literally" would apply to bulk compounding).

[38] See W. States, 535 U.S. at 362.

[39] Id.

[40] Statement of Steven K. Galson, Acting Director, Center for Drug Evaluation and Research, U.S. Food and Drug Administration, before the Senate Committee on Health, Education, Labor and Pensions, Hearing on "Federal and State Role in Pharmacy Compounding and Reconstitution: Exploring the Right Mix to Protect Patients," (October 23, 2003). See also Western States, 535 U.S. at 369 ("...it would not make sense to require compounded drugs created to meet the unique needs of patients to undergo the testing required for the new drug approval process. Pharmacists do not make enough money from small-scale compounding to make safety and efficacy testing of their compounded drugs economically feasible, so requiring such testing would force pharmacists to stop providing compounded drugs.")

[41] W. States, 535 U.S. at 369.

[42] Id. at 368-69.

[43] 21 U.S.C. §355.

[44] W. States, 535 U.S. at 370.

[45] P.L. 87-781, 76 Stat. 780 (1962) (current version as amended at 21 U.S.C. §§301-392).

[46] Id.; see generally Bryan Christopher Moody, "Prescription Medication and Consumer Protection: A Time for Reform," The Journal of Pharmacy & Law, vol. 5 (1996), p. 21 ("Additionally, the Drug Amendments of 1962 required the following: that drug companies register with the FDA and be inspected by the FDA every two years, that all drug company records be made available for inspection, that adverse drug reactions be transmitted to the FDA, that the FDA be given full authority to regulate the advertising of prescription drugs and all advertising must relate to the adverse effects and contraindications to consumer, and that investigational drug studies require informed patient consent prior to trials on humans.")

[47] See 21 U.S.C. §360(g)(1).

[48] See 21 U.S.C. §374(a)(2)(A).

[49] See Wedgewood Vill. Pharm., Inc. v. United States, 421 F.3d 263, 269 (3d Cir. 2005) (holding that a compounder was not exempt from non-record inspections under 21 U.S.C. §374(a)).

[50] P.L. 105-115, 111 Stat. 2296 (1997). The FDAMA was a product of a 1992 FDA Compliance Policy Guide that outlined the agency's policies regarding drug compounding. See W. States., 535 U.S. at 362-64 ("Congress turned portions of this policy into law when it enacted the FDAMA in 1997).

[51] CPG §7132.16 (Mar. 1992).

[52] W. States, 535 U.S. at 362.

[53] S.Rept. 105-43, Committee on Labor and Human Resources, p. 67 (July 1, 1997).

[54] See 21 U.S.C. §353a(a).

[55] Id. (citing Sections 501(a)(2)(B) (adulteration), 502(f)(1) (misbranding), 505 (new drugs)).

[56] 21 U.S.C. §353a(a).

[57] 21 U.S.C. §§353a(b)(1)(A)-(C).

[58] 21 U.S.C. §353a(b)(1)(D). The definition of the term "inordinate amounts" is delegated in the statute to the Secretary of Health and Human Services. Id. FDA regulations have not yet formally defined the term "inordinate amounts." See 21 C.F.R. §216.23 et seq.

[59] 21 U.S.C. §353a(b)(3)(A).

[60] 21 U.S.C. §353a(b)(3)(B).

[61] 21 U.S.C. §353a(c).

[62] 535 U.S. at 360.

[63] See Alaska Airlines, Inc. v. Brock, 480 U.S. 678, 684 (1987) (internal quotations and citations omitted).

[64] Compare W. State Med Ctr. v. Shalala, 238 F.3d 1090, 1096-98 (9th Cir. 2001), aff'd on other grounds, 535 U.S. 357 (2002), with Medical Ctr. Pharmacy v. Mukasey, 536 F.3d 383, 401(5th Cir. 2008). The Supreme Court in Western States declined to rule on the issue of severability. 535 U.S. at 366 ("Because neither party petitioned for certiorari on the severability issue, we have no occasion to review that portion of the Court of Appeals decision.") For a more in depth discussion on these two cases and the resulting circuit split, see CRS Report R40503, FDA's Authority to Regulate Drug Compounding: A Legal Analysis, by Jennifer Staman.

[65] The Ninth Circuit Court of Appeals covers the states of Alaska, Arizona, California, Idaho, Montana, Nevada, Oregon, Washington, and Hawaii. See 28 U.S.C. §41.

[66] W. State Med Ctr., 238 F.3d at 1096-98.

[67] Medical Ctr. Pharmacy, 536 F.3d at 401. The Fifth Circuit's jurisdiction is limited to the states of Louisiana, Mississippi, and Texas. See 28 U.S.C. §41.

[68] An unpublished federal district court decision in Colorado, faced with both parties in agreement that the FDAMA's advertising provisions were severable from the rest of the act, opined that the Fifth Circuit's decision with respect to severability was not "so palpably incorrect that applying its rule would be clearly be error." See United States v. Bader, No. 07-CR-338, 2009 WL 2219258 at *9 (D. Colo. July 23, 2009), aff'd 678 F.3d 858 (11th Cir. 2012). On appeal to the Tenth Circuit, the appellate court found the Fifth Circuit's decision to be inapplicable to the case at hand as the case did not implicate any provisions of the FDAMA. 678 F.3d at 888-89 ("Consequently, Medical Center Pharmacy is inapposite.")

[69] Compliance Policy Guide §460.200 (May 29, 2002).

[70] Wedgewood Vill. Pharm., Inc. v. United States, 421 F.3d 263, 272 (3d Cir. 2005).

[71] Bader, 678 F.3d at 888 (noting that the "overarching premise of [the 2002 CPG on compounding] was that, generally, the FDA had maintained some degree of regulatory authority over pharmacy compounding both before Western States ... and the FDAMA").

[72] CPG §460.200 (May 29, 2002); see generally United States v. Livdahl, 459 F. Supp. 2d 1255, 1263 (S.D. Fla. 2005) (noting that "in the wake of Western States, the FDA issued a new [CPG] dealing with compounded drugs [similar to the one codified in the FDAMA] ... [t]his new policy is unaffected by the decision in Western States).

[73] See Food and Drug Administration, "Medical Center Pharmacy v. Mukasey," press release, May 6, 2009, http://www.fda.gov/Drugs/GuidanceComplianceRegulatoryInformation/PharmacyCompounding/ucm134919.htm ("In the meantime, FDA will follow the court's decision in the Fifth Circuit and with respect to the plaintiffs covered by the decision. Elsewhere, the agency will continue to follow the enforcement approach reflected in the Compliance Policy Guide (CPG) section 460.200 [Pharmacy Compounding] issued by FDA on May 29, 2002."); see also Letter from Alonza E. Cruse, Director, Los Angeles District, U.S. Food and Drug Administration, to Ari S. Schafer, Civic Center Pharmacy (December 16, 2008), available at http://www.fda.gov/ICECI/EnforcementActions/ WarningLetters/ 2008/ ucm1048048.htm; see also Letter from Alonza E. Cruse, Director, Los Angeles District, U.S. Food and Drug Administration, to Charles T. Bonner, Steven's Pharmacy (November 12, 2008), available at http://www.fda.gov/ ICECI/EnforcementActions/ WarningLetters/2008/ucm1048074.htm.

[74] The practical effect of whether the FDAMA's compounding provisions apply or whether the CPG applies is not readily apparent, as both the compounding provisions of the FDAMA and the CPG are rooted in authority provided by the FDCA. Compare 21 U.S.C. §503A(a) (stating that Sections 501(a)(2)(B), 502(f)(1) and 505 of the FDCA do not apply to certain

compounding activity) with CPG §460.200 (May 29, 2002) (providing guidance on "what types of compounding might be subject to enforcement action under current law").

[75] CPG §460.200 (May 29, 2002).

[76] Id.

[77] Id.

[78] Id.

[79] For a more in depth discussion on the 2002 FDA CPG on compounding, see CRS Report R40503, FDA's Authority to Regulate Drug Compounding: A Legal Analysis, by Jennifer Staman.

[80] See CPG §608.400 (July 14, 2003). The FDAMA's provision on compounding addressed human, not animal, use. See 21 U.S.C. §353a(a).

[81] See CPG §608.400 (July 14, 2003).

[82] Id. The "new animal drug" provisions of the FDCA are similar, but not identical, to the provisions for human drugs. Pursuant to Section 512 of the FDCA, absent FDA approval, a "new animal drug" is "deemed unsafe, which, in turn, renders the drug "adulterated" under Section 501(a) and "misbranded" under Section 502(f) unless the drug bears "adequate directions for use." See 21 U.S.C. §360b. Hence, similar "to human drugs, any drug ... the composition of which has not already been approved by the FDA constitutes a 'new animal drug' within the meaning of the statute.'" See Medical Ctr. Pharm., 536 F.3d at 407 (internal citations omitted).

[83] See CPG §460.200 (May 29, 2002); see also CPG §608.400 (July 14, 2003).

[84] Id.

[85] Id. While animal drug compounding is beyond the scope of this report, the overlap in the legal framework for human and animal drugs, see supra footnote 82, make the FDA's 2003 guidance useful to gauge the agency's general approach toward the regulation of drug compounding.

[86] Id.

[87] Id.

[88] See CPG §460.200 (May 29, 2002). The CPG, as a general policy statement, as opposed to a rule that affords the public notice and an opportunity to comment on the rule, does not have the force of law,88 and does not receive the fullest deference from courts of law. See United States v. Mead Corp., 533 U.S. 218, 229 (2001). Instead, a CPG "merely provide[s] guidance for FDA agents in determining possible violations, within their discretion." Professionals & Patients for Customized Care v. Shalala, 847 F. Supp. 1359, 1365 (S.D. Tex. 1994). For a lengthier discussion of the legal effect of the CPG, see CRS Report R40503, FDA's Authority to Regulate Drug Compounding: A Legal Analysis, by Jennifer Staman.

[89] 21 U.S.C. §353a(a) (exempting certain compounding activities from the reach of the FDCA Sections 501(a)(2)(B) (adulteration), 502(f)(1) (misbranding), 505 (new drugs)); but see Medical Ctr. Pharm., 536 F.3d at 405 (noting that because Congress started from a default premise that the FDCA's "adulteration, misbranding, and new drug provisions apply to – and thereby restrict – all drugs created by any means," including compounding, that the FDCA must reach compounding). However, it can be argued that the understanding of a future Congress regarding previously enacted legislation will "rarely override a reasonable interpretation of a statute that can be gleaned from its language." See Consumer Prod. Safety Comm'n v. GTE Sylvania, Inc., 447 U.S. 102, 118 n.13 (1980).

[90] Brief of the Appellant United States, United States v. Franck's Lab, Inc., 11-15350-BB (11th Cir 2012). at pg. 26.

[91] Food and Drug Administration, "Is It Really FDA Approved?," press release, February 20, 2009, http://www.fda.gov/downloads/ForConsumers/ConsumerUpdates/UCM143301.pdf.

[92] Brief of the Appellant United States, United States v. Franck's Lab, Inc., 11-15350-BB (11th Cir 2012). at pg. 26; see also Professionals & Patients for Customized Care v. Shalala, 56 F.3d 592, 593-594 (5th Cir. 1995).

[93] Medical Ctr. Pharm., 536 F.3d at 399.

[94] Id.

[95] See W. States Med. Ctr., 535 U.S. at 369 ("[R]equiring such testing would force pharmacists to stop providing compounded drugs.")

[96] See generally Franck's Lab, 816 F. Supp. 2d at 1235-1239 (discussing the cases that have examined the scope of the FDA's authority with respect to compounding).

[97] Id.; see also Med. Ctr. Pharm., 536 F.3d at 399 ("Construing the FDCA to give the FDA authority over compounding would thus not necessarily 'lead to a result so bizarre that Congress could not have intended it.'")(internal citations omitted); In re Wedgewood Vill. Pharmacy, 270 F. Supp. 2d 525, 549 (D.N.J. 2003) ("Congress intended that the FDCA, both in its original form and as amended, allow the FDA broad enforcement powers to fulfill its mandate that it protect the public from unsafe medication.")

[98] Franck's Lab, 816 F. Supp. 2d at 1246.

[99] See Wedgewood Vill. Pharm, 421 F.3d at 272 ("We agree that the factors set forth in the CPG are reasonable and that they reflect the FDA's 'careful consideration ... over a long period of time.") (internal citations omitted).

[100] See Franck's Lab, 816 F. Supp. 2d at 1239.

[101] The plain language of a statute is the starting point for statutory interpretation, and if a statute's terms are "plain," the Supreme Court has noted that a court should look no further and enforce the law "according to its terms." See Hartford Underwriters Ins. Co. v. Union Planters Bank, N.A., 530 U.S. 1, 6 (2000).

[102] 21 U.S.C. §355(a).

[103] 21 U.S.C. §351(a)(1)(B).

[104] 21 U.S.C. §352(f)(1).

[105] Medical Ctr. Pharm., 536 F.3d at 395.

[106] Id.; see also United States v. 9/1 Kg. Containers, 854 F.2d 173, 176 (7th Cir. 1988) (holding, with respect to the misbranding provisions of the FFDCA, "Congress gave the FDA comprehensive powers to license the manufacture of drugs and limit theirs sales," leaving it to the discretion of the FDA to regulate bulk compounding); United States v. Algon Chemical, Inc., 879 F.2d 1154, 1163 (3d Cir. 1989) (concluding that Congress did not intend that bulk drug compounding "be excluded from the Act's labeling requirements").

[107] 21 U.S.C. §360b(j).

[108] Medical Ctr. Pharm., 536 F.3d at 395; but see Franck's Lab, 816 F. Supp. 2d at 1244 ("However, if we were to presume a delegation of power from the absence of an express withholding of such power, agencies would enjoy virtually limitless hegemony") (internal citations and quotations omitted).

[109] Id. at 398 (summarizing the pharmacists' position); see also Franck's Lab, 816 F. Supp. 2d at 1243-44.

[110] See Whitman v. American Trucking Assoc., 531 U.S. 457, 458 (2001) ("[Congress] does not, one might say, hide elephants in mouseholes"); see also FDA v. Brown & Williamson Tobacco Corp., 529 U.S. 120, 160 ("[W]e are confident that Congress could not have intended to delegate a decision of such economic and political significance to an agency in so cryptic a fashion.")

[111] Franck's Lab, 816 F. Supp. 2d at 1245-46.

[112] Food, Drugs and Comsetis: Hearings Before a Cubcomm. of the Comm. on Commerce, 74 Cong. 100, 102 (1935) (statement of Robert P. Fischelis, president American Pharmaceutical Ass'n).

[113] See generally Crandon v. United States, 494 U.S. 152, 160 (1990).

[114] See generally Franck's Lab, 816 F. Supp. 2d at 1235-1239 (discussing the cases that have examined the scope of the FDA's authority with respect to compounding).

[115] See Gonzales v. Raich, 545 U.S. 1, 22 (2005) (holding that the authority under the Commerce Clause extends such that Congress can regulate activities when, taken in the aggregate, substantially affect interstate commerce).

[116] But see Franck's Lab, 816 F. Supp. 2d at 1214 ("[T]he FDA has taken the bright-line position that any compounding of animal medications from bulk substances violates ... the FDCA ...")

[117] See CPG §460.200 (May 29, 2002); see also CPG §608.400 (July 14, 2003).

[118] This lack of resolution could be a considerable burden on traditional compounders, whose conduct could be in violation of federal law. As one court noted, "it remains no small burden for compounding pharmacists ... to 'live in sin,' [as] their livelihood [has] no greater assurance than the FDA's good graces." See Medical Ctr. Pharm., 536 F.3d at 399-400.

[119] See, e.g., Wedgewood Vill. Pharm., 421 F.3d at 272-73.

In: Drug Compounding
Editor: Martti Bram
ISBN: 978-1-63117-360-8

Chapter 3

DRUG COMPOUNDING: CLEAR AUTHORITY AND MORE RELIABLE DATA NEEDED TO STRENGTHEN FDA OVERSIGHT*

United States Government Accountability Office

WHY GAO DID THIS STUDY

Drug compounding is the process by which a pharmacist combines, mixes, or alters ingredients to create a drug tailored to the medical needs of an individual. An outbreak of fungal meningitis in 2012 linked to contaminated compounded drugs has raised concerns about state and federal oversight of drug compounding. GAO was asked to update its 2003 testimony on drug compounding. Specifically, this report addresses (1) the status of FDA's authority to oversee drug compounding, and the gaps, if any, between state and federal authority; (2) how FDA has used its data and authority to oversee drug compounding; and (3) the actions taken or planned by states or national pharmacy organizations to improve oversight of drug compounding. GAO reviewed relevant statutes and guidance; reviewed FDA data; and interviewed officials from FDA, national pharmacy organizations, and four states with varied geography, population, and pharmacy regulations.

* This is an edited, reformatted and augmented version of the United States Government Accountability Office publication, No. GAO-13-702, dated July 2013.

What GAO Recommends

To help ensure that the entities that compound drugs have appropriate oversight, Congress should consider clarifying FDA's authority to oversee drug compounding. In addition, FDA should ensure its databases collect reliable and timely data on inspections associated with compounded drugs, and differentiate drug compounders from manufacturers. HHS's comments support the need to clarify FDA's authority, and stated that the information in its inspection database could be improved and that it would consider whether it can differentiate compounding pharmacies from manufacturers.

What GAO Found

The authority of the Food and Drug Administration (FDA), an agency within the Department of Health and Human Services (HHS), to oversee drug compounding is unclear. Two federal circuit court decisions have resulted in differing FDA authority in different parts of the country. According to FDA officials, these inconsistent decisions and the agency's limited inspection authority over pharmacies have created challenges in FDA's ability to inspect and take enforcement action against entities engaging in drug compounding. For example, from 2002 through 2012, in order to inspect some facilities engaged in drug compounding, FDA officials said they had to obtain 11 warrants to gain access to drug compounders' facilities that had challenged FDA's inspection authority. GAO also found that while FDA and national pharmacy organization officials generally agreed that states regulate the practice of pharmacy and FDA regulates drug manufacturing, there was no consensus on whether compounding drugs in large quantities—in anticipation of individual prescriptions or without prescriptions—and selling those drugs across state lines falls within the practice of pharmacy or is a type of drug manufacturing that should be overseen by FDA. This lack of consensus and differing FDA authority to oversee compounded drugs across the country has resulted in gaps in oversight of drug compounding.

FDA lacks timely and reliable information to oversee the entities that compound drugs, but has found problems through its limited oversight. Specifically, FDA's inspection database cannot identify all of the agency's inspections of compounding pharmacies, or the final classification of inspection results, for all of the inspections. Until 2013, FDA limited its inspections of compounding pharmacies to those conducted in response to complaints or adverse events. However, the agency recently inspected compounding pharmacies that it identified as posing a significant threat to public health from poor sterile drug production practices in the past and found problems, such as concerns about a lack of sterility, which resulted in recalls of compounded drugs. In addition, drug manufacturers are required to register with FDA and are subject to FDA's inspection and drug approval processes; pharmacies meeting certain requirements are generally exempt from registration. However, some compounding pharmacies may have registered with FDA to market themselves as "FDA-registered" which may lead some purchasers to assume that FDA has inspected or approved their compounded drugs; whereas, according to FDA officials, this is generally not the case.

The states GAO reviewed—California, Connecticut, Florida, and Iowa—have each taken actions to enhance their oversight of drug compounding. For example, Florida required all pharmacies—both those located in the state and out-of-state that sell drugs in Florida—to notify the board of their compounding activities. In addition, national pharmacy organizations have undertaken efforts to help states oversee drug compounding. For example, a national pharmacy organization is working with Iowa to inspect out-of-state pharmacies that ship drugs into the state. However, according to national pharmacy organizations and officials from state boards of pharmacy, some states do not have the resources to inspect pharmacies on a regular basis. Instead, these states inspect pharmacies only in response to a complaint or a reported adverse drug event.

ABBREVIATIONS

FACTS	Field Accomplishments and Compliance Tracking System
FDA	Food and Drug Administration
FDAMA	Food and Drug Administration Modernization Act of 1997
FDCA	Federal Food, Drug, and Cosmetic Act
HHS	Department of Health and Human Services
NABP	National Association of Boards of Pharmacy
OIG	Office of Inspector General
PCAB	Pharmacy Compounding Accreditation Board
USP	The United States Pharmacopeial Convention

July 31, 2013
The Honorable Elijah Cummings
Ranking Member
Committee on Oversight and Government Reform
House of Representatives

The Honorable John Tierney
Ranking Member
Subcommittee on National Security
Committee on Oversight and Government Reform
House of Representatives

Drug compounding is the process by which a pharmacist or doctor combines, mixes, or alters ingredients to create a drug tailored to the medical needs of an individual patient. Compounding, a traditional component of the practice of pharmacy, is typically used to prepare drugs that are not commercially available, such as a drug for a patient who is allergic to an ingredient in a mass-produced pharmaceutical product.[1] Traditionally, state pharmacy regulatory bodies (e.g., boards of pharmacy) regulate pharmacy practice, including drug compounding activities, through state laws and regulations. The Food and Drug Administration (FDA) is the agency within the Department of Health and Human Services (HHS) responsible for assuring the safety and effectiveness of drugs marketed in the United States.[2] Under the Federal Food, Drug, and Cosmetic Act (FDCA), and its implementing regulations, FDA approves new drugs and regulates the manufacture, marketing, and distribution of pharmaceutical products.[3]

An outbreak of fungal meningitis in 2012 linked to contaminated compounded drugs—resulting in over 60 deaths and hundreds of people becoming ill—has led to questions about the safety and quality of compounded drugs, and raised concerns about state and federal oversight of drug compounding.[4] Concerns have also been raised by FDA and others, including members of Congress and public health advocates, that some pharmacies are going beyond traditional drug compounding by producing large quantities of compounded drugs without prescriptions for individual patients, and selling those compounded drugs to facilities in multiple states. Many believe that these types of pharmacies are manufacturing drugs under the guise of compounding without meeting safety and other requirements with which drug manufacturers must comply.

You asked us to update our 2003 testimony on drug compounding. 5 Specifically, this report addresses (1) the status of FDA's authority to oversee drug compounding, and the gaps, if any, between state and federal authority to oversee drug compounding; (2) how FDA has used its data and authority to oversee drug compounding; and (3) the actions taken or planned by states or national pharmacy organizations to improve oversight of drug compounding.

To describe the status of FDA's authority to oversee drug compounding and any gaps between state and federal authority, we reviewed FDCA provisions pertaining to drug compounding and other relevant federal statutes, regulations, and guidance documents on federal oversight of drug compounding, including FDA's 2002 compliance policy guide on drug compounding. We also reviewed other relevant FDA documents, and interviewed FDA officials on any gaps or proposed actions to address gaps, or to clarify federal and state authority. We selected four states— California, Connecticut, Florida, and Iowa—and reviewed documents, and interviewed officials from state regulatory bodies in each of these states. 6 (App. I contains information on the four states.) In addition, we reviewed documents, and interviewed officials from national organizations representing pharmacies and pharmacists—including the American Pharmacists Association, American Society of Health-System Pharmacists, International Academy of Compounding Pharmacists, and National Community Pharmacists Association—and other organizations, including the National Association of Boards of Pharmacy (NABP) and the United States Pharmacopeial Convention (USP).[7] We also reviewed reports and studies related to oversight of drug compounding, and interviewed officials involved in those studies, including those from the Congressional Research Service and the HHS Office of Inspector General (OIG).

To examine how FDA has used its data and authority to oversee drug compounding, we reviewed documents and interviewed FDA officials—including officials in the Center for Drug Evaluation and Research, Office of Regulatory Affairs, and Office of the Chief Counsel—regarding data FDA collects on compounded drugs, the entities that compound them, and FDA inspections of those entities. Specifically, we examined data related to drug compounding from (1) FDA's Drug Registration and Listing System on entities that compound drugs that registered with FDA in its drug manufacturer database, and (2) FDA's Field Accomplishments and Compliance Tracking System (FACTS) on inspections of entities that compound drugs. We also interviewed FDA officials on the availability and limitations of FDA's data on adverse events associated with compounded drugs. We compared FDA's data on compounded drugs and the entities that compound them, including FDA's inspections and outcomes of those inspections, to standards described in *Standards for Internal Control in the Federal Government*—which specifies that relevant, reliable, and timely information be available for management decision making and external reporting purposes.[8]

We also reviewed information on FDA's efforts in 2013 to conduct inspections of entities that, according to the agency, were known to have produced sterile compounded drugs in the past. To assess the reliability of the FDA data, we reviewed FDA guidance and related documentation; interviewed knowledgeable agency officials; and viewed data FDA made available from these databases on its website. We determined that the data were sufficiently reliable for purposes of our report.

To identify actions planned or taken by states or national pharmacy organizations, we reviewed state laws and regulations, and proposed changes to state laws and regulations, in the four states we selected. For each state, we reviewed documents and interviewed representatives of the states' pharmacy regulatory bodies regarding actions taken or planned relating to the oversight of drug compounding, the implications of existing and proposed state laws and regulations, and the challenges state regulatory bodies face in overseeing drug compounding.

We also discussed the states' pharmacy inspection and enforcement activities, as well as state efforts to collect pharmacy data. In addition, we reviewed surveys of states—for example, results of surveys of states to determine the number requiring compliance with USP provisions for sterile compounding.

We also reviewed documents and interviewed officials from national pharmacy organizations, including NABP, regarding the actions planned or taken by these national pharmacy organizations related to the oversight of drug compounding.

We conducted this performance audit from February 2013 to July 2013 in accordance with generally accepted government auditing standards. Those standards require that we plan and perform the audit to obtain sufficient, appropriate evidence to provide a reasonable basis for our findings and conclusions based on our audit objectives. We believe that the evidence obtained provides a reasonable basis for our findings and conclusions based on our audit objectives.

BACKGROUND

Drug Compounding by Pharmacies

Traditionally, a drug is compounded, through the process of mixing, combining, or altering ingredients, to create a customized drug tailored to the medical needs of an individual patient upon receipt of a prescription. For example, a pharmacist may tailor a drug for a patient who is allergic to an ingredient in a manufactured drug or prepare a liquid formulation for a patient who has difficulty swallowing pills. Some pharmacies also compound drugs in advance of receiving individual patient prescriptions in anticipation of receiving prescriptions based on historical prescribing patterns, a practice referred to as anticipatory compounding. Compounded drugs include nonsterile preparations, such as capsules, ointments, creams, gels, and suppositories; and sterile preparations, including intravenously administered fluids and injectable drugs. Compounded sterile drugs pose special risks of contamination if not made properly and require special safeguards to prevent injury or death to patients receiving them.

Drug compounding is an integral part of the pharmacy profession and is practiced in a variety of settings, including hospital pharmacies, community pharmacies, chain drug store pharmacies, and home infusion settings. The exact proportion of all prescriptions filled by compounded drugs is unknown. In 2003, we reported that estimates ranged from 1 percent to 10 percent.[9] More recently, in 2013, the International Academy of Compounding Pharmacists estimated that the compounding industry made up 1 to 3 percent of the U.S. prescription drug market.

The exact number of pharmacies that compound drugs is also unknown. In 2013, the International Academy of Compounding Pharmacists provided the following estimates:

- About 26,000 community-based pharmacies reported that they provide some sort of prescription compounding services, based on information from the National Council of Prescription Drug Program's database on pharmacies.
- Of those 26,000 community-based pharmacies, about 7,500 pharmacies specialize in compounding.
- Of those 7,500 community-based pharmacies that specialize in compounding, about 3,000 pharmacies compound both sterile and nonsterile preparations.

- In addition, there are about 8,200 hospital pharmacies in the United States, and all of them are likely conducting some sort of compounding, both sterile and nonsterile.

A recent report indicates that there has been an increase in the outsourcing of drug compounding in the last decade, primarily by hospitals. In April 2013, the HHS-OIG reported that nearly all (92 percent) of surveyed hospitals that participated in Medicare reported using compounded sterile products, and that more than three-fourths of these hospitals (77 percent) purchased some of these compounded drugs from at least one outside pharmacy.[10] The HHS-OIG found factors that hospitals cited for outsourcing included the need to ensure a ready supply of products in the event of shortages and the need for products with extended shelf lives, which require sophisticated equipment and testing to prepare these products that may not be readily available on the hospital premises.

State Regulation of Pharmacy Practice

State pharmacy regulatory bodies are responsible for oversight of the practice of pharmacy. All 50 states describe drug compounding in their state laws and regulations on pharmacy practice, although specific statutes or regulations vary across states, according to NABP.

USP is involved in setting standards that affect compounding.[11] According to USP, compounding standards help practitioners adhere to widely acknowledged, scientifically sound procedures and best practices, and facilitate the delivery of consistent and good-quality prepared medicines to patients. Twenty-five state pharmacy regulatory bodies reported that they require compliance with USP's chapter on sterile compounding, according to the NABP's 2013 survey of pharmacy law.[12]

FDA Regulation of Drug Compounding

FDA considers compounded drugs to be "new drugs" subject to FDA oversight; however, the agency has acknowledged that it is not practicable for pharmacies to complete and obtain approval for a new drug application for each compounded drug prepared for an individual patient.[13] In 1992, FDA, through guidance, and, in 1997, Congress, through legislation, attempted to clarify when compounded drugs will be exempt from certain requirements of the FDCA, including new drug approval requirements. Specifically, the Food and Drug Administration Modernization Act of 1997 (FDAMA) enacted section 503A of the FDCA. This section exempted drug products compounded by a pharmacist or physician based on a valid prescription for a compounded product that is necessary for the identified patient from three key provisions of the FDCA that are otherwise applicable to drugs, provided the pharmacy had, among other conditions, not solicited prescriptions or advertised or promoted the compounded drugs.[14]

In 2001, however, the United States Court of Appeals for the Ninth Circuit struck down all of the advertising, promotion, and solicitation provisions of section 503A of the FDCA because those provisions violated the Free Speech Clause of the First Amendment. The court also held that, because these provisions could not be severed from the remainder of section 503A, all of section 503A was invalid. In 2002, the United States Supreme Court struck down the law's advertising, promotion, and solicitation restrictions without addressing whether the rest of section 503A remained law. As a result, FDA issued a revised version of its compliance policy guide on drug compounding in 2002, which provides guidance, in light of the Ninth Circuit and Supreme Court decisions, on the types of factors the agency will consider in determining whether to take enforcement action against drug compounders for violations of the FDCA. These factors include activities, such as offering compounded drug products at wholesale, that suggest a drug compounder is engaged in drug manufacturing, rather than drug compounding. Subsequently, in 2005, the United States Court of Appeals for the Fifth Circuit issued a decision holding that, although section 503A's advertising, promotion, and solicitation restrictions were invalid, these restrictions could be severed from the rest of section 503A and, therefore, the law's remaining drug compounding provisions remain valid. See appendix II for details about these developments and how they have affected FDA's authority to oversee drug compounding.

The FDCA provides FDA authority to inspect pharmacies that compound drugs; however, this authority is limited. Generally, FDA's inspection authority does not extend to a pharmacy's records if the pharmacy meets certain requirements.[15] While FDA has not routinely inspected compounding pharmacies, FDA has used its authority to conduct some inspections in recent years, generally in response to complaints. These inspections have resulted in FDA issuing inspection observation reports, which are called FDA form 483s, and, in some cases, warning letters.[16] FDA's FACTS database contains information on these inspections, including the type of inspection (e.g., routine or in response to a complaint).

Under the FDCA, drug manufacturers are required to register with FDA and list the drugs they manufacture.[17] The FDCA exempts from these registration and listing requirements those pharmacies that meet certain requirements.[18] FDA's Drug Registration and Listing System contains information on drug establishments that have registered with FDA to market their drugs in the United States. These establishments provide information, including company name and address, and identify the drugs they manufacture for commercial distribution in the United States.

UNCLEAR FEDERAL AUTHORITY AND LACK OF CONSENSUS ON WHEN DRUG COMPOUNDING BECOMES MANUFACTURING

Although FDAMA attempted to clarify FDA's authority to oversee drug compounding, subsequent court decisions have contributed to a lack of clarity regarding the legal standards FDA must apply to oversee drug compounding. Specifically, two federal circuit court decisions resulted in differing FDA authority over drug compounding in different parts of the country, which has affected FDA's ability to oversee drug compounding. Section 503A provisions exempting certain compounded drugs from the FDCA's good manufacturing practice, certain labeling, and new drug and abbreviated new drug application requirements are in effect in those states in the Fifth Circuit, in which the U.S. Court of Appeals has held that the law, other than its advertising, promotion, and solicitation provisions, is valid. However, FDA follows its 2002 compliance policy guide in states in the Ninth Circuit, in which the U.S. Court of Appeals has held all of the drug compounding provisions in section 503A are invalid. In states outside of the Fifth and Ninth Circuits, where federal courts have not considered the validity of these drug compounding provisions, FDA considers both section 503A's drug compounding provisions and its 2002 compliance policy guide to guide its oversight. Figure 1 shows how FDA generally conducts its oversight of drug compounding in different parts of the country based on the differing court decisions.

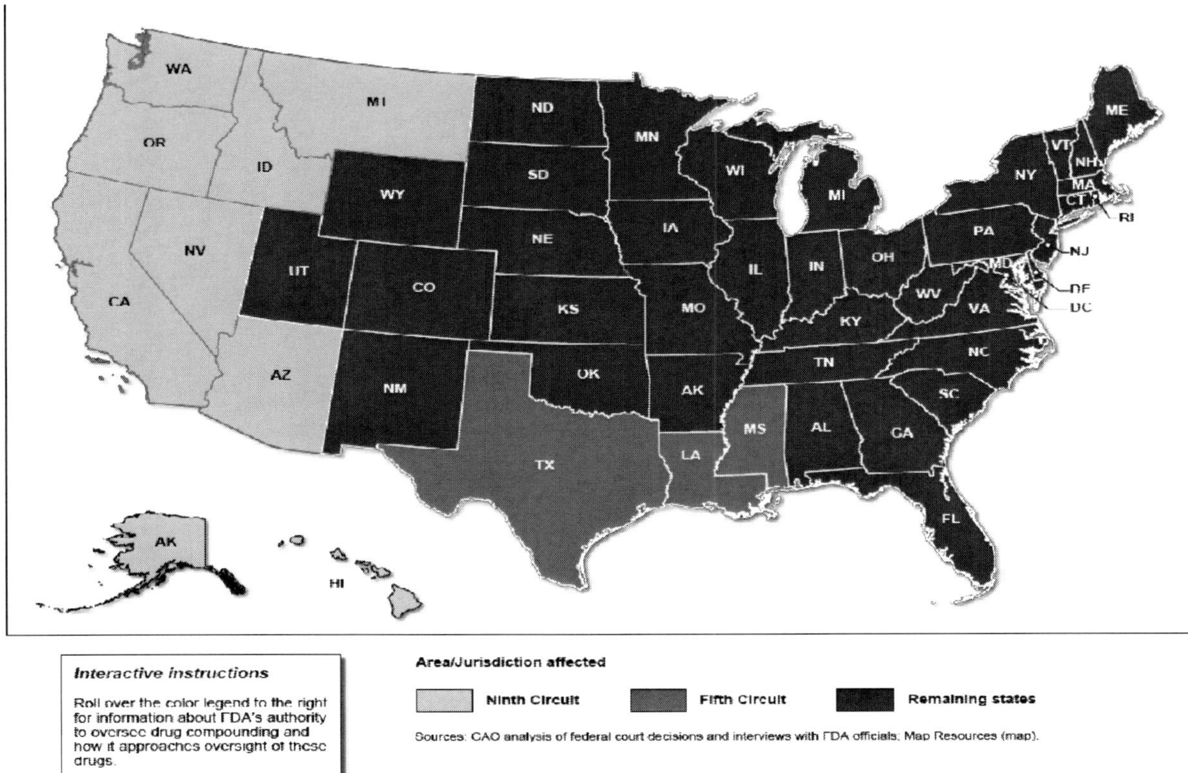

Figure 1. Food and Drug Administration (FDA) Oversight of Drug Compounding.

Furthermore, according to FDA officials, the agency's inconsistent authority to oversee drug compounding and the agency's limited inspection authority over pharmacies have led to legal challenges to FDA's authority to inspect entities engaging in drug compounding and to take appropriate enforcement actions against these entities. For example, from 2002 through 2012, FDA had to obtain 11 inspection warrants to gain access to drug compounders' facilities and records, representing nearly half of the 25 administrative warrants obtained by FDA for all FDA-regulated products in that same period, according to agency officials.[19] FDA officials said that these entities refused FDA access to their facilities or records, citing the provision of the FDCA that limits the agency's inspection authority over a pharmacy that is in compliance with state and local laws.[20] FDA officials added that if the agency is required to obtain a warrant before gaining access, the agency may be delayed in its efforts to curb an outbreak or take enforcement action and the entity may have time to clean up its facility or alter its records to avoid enforcement action. FDA officials also said that if the agency finds significant issues during an inspection of a drug compounder, to determine whether to take action against the compounder the agency must first consider its legal authority in the particular jurisdiction in which the compounder operates and whether any FDA action is likely to be challenged in court. According to FDA officials, engaging in this type of analysis may have resulted in a long lag time between the inspection and the issuance of a warning letter.

In addition, we found a lack of consensus regarding when drug compounding becomes drug manufacturing. Officials from FDA and national pharmacy organizations we interviewed generally agreed that traditional drug compounding involves a patient-specific prescription for a customized medication that is not otherwise commercially available, and there was agreement that this type of compounding is part of the practice of pharmacy and generally overseen by the states. Further, there was agreement that FDA has clear authority to oversee drug manufacturing and drug manufacturers. However, there was not agreement on whether compounding pharmacies that are engaged in large-scale drug compounding, producing these drugs in anticipation of individual prescriptions or without prescriptions, and selling them across state lines, are engaged in the practice of pharmacy or are engaged in drug manufacturing. As a result, there is a lack of consensus regarding whether states should have primary responsibility for regulating these entities as pharmacies, or FDA should have primary responsibility to regulate them as manufacturers. This lack of consensus on who has primary responsibility to regulate entities engaged in these practices and differing FDA authority applicable to compounded drugs across the country has resulted in gaps in oversight of drug compounding.

Further, according to officials from FDA and most of the organizations we spoke with, the line is not clear when anticipatory compounding is part of the practice of pharmacy and when anticipatory compounding crosses into drug manufacturing. For example, officials from one national pharmacy organization said that if a certain number of patients come to a pharmacy every month for progesterone suppositories and the pharmacy makes enough for a month's supply in advance based on the history of these prescriptions, then a pharmacy's compounding of the drug in advance should be considered drug compounding and not manufacturing. However, these officials added that a pharmacy that makes 10,000 sterile compounded injectables in advance of a prescription and ships them across 18 states may be engaged in manufacturing.

Noting this lack of clarity regarding when drug compounding becomes manufacturing, FDA has been working on a proposal that would create a new category of "nontraditional compounding," which would be subject to FDA oversight. According to congressional testimony and public statements,[21] FDA's new category of "nontraditional drug compounders" would fall between traditional drug compounding and drug manufacturing. FDA officials said they believe this new category would subject entities with a higher potential to adversely affect a large number of patients to appropriate and effective FDA regulation and oversight. FDA's proposal describes an entity as engaging in nontraditional compounding if it produces sterile compounded products in advance of or without an individual patient prescription, and ships these sterile compounded products across state lines. Under FDA's proposal, state pharmacy regulatory bodies would continue to have primary responsibility to oversee traditional drug compounding and FDA would have express statutory authority to oversee this new category of nontraditional drug compounding.[22]

Some national pharmacy organizations said that the creation of a new category of nontraditional drug compounding is not necessary because they believe drug compounding and drug manufacturing are already distinct. For example, officials from one national pharmacy organization we interviewed said the establishment of a new category of nontraditional drug compounding could create more confusion between drug compounding and manufacturing, unless this new category is carefully crafted. These officials said that states should regulate drug compounding and FDA should regulate drug manufacturing, and that once an entity crosses the line between drug compounding and manufacturing, there should be a seamless handoff from the state to FDA. However, other organizations we spoke with generally agreed with FDA's proposed tiered system and said that entities in this new category should be regulated by FDA, not by state pharmacy regulatory bodies.

FDA LACKS RELIABLE AND TIMELY DATA ON COMPOUNDING PHARMACIES, BUT HAS FOUND PROBLEMS THROUGH ITS LIMITED OVERSIGHT

FDA lacks reliable information on entities that compound drugs, the types of drugs being compounded, and adverse events related to compounded drugs. Until 2013, FDA limited its inspections of compounding pharmacies to those conducted in response to complaints or adverse events, called "for cause" inspections; however, the agency has recently conducted inspections of compounding pharmacies that were known to produce "high-risk" sterile compounded drugs, and identified serious problems.

FDA Has Not Collected Reliable and Timely Data on Compounded Drugs and the Entities That Prepare Them

FDA officials, including the FDA Commissioner, have stated that, under the FDCA, compounding pharmacies are generally not required to register with FDA or list their products, and therefore FDA does not know who they are and what they are compounding.[23] As a result, FDA has stated that one of the reasons it has not routinely inspected compounding pharmacies is because the agency does not know who they are.

Officials with some of the organizations we interviewed said there has been confusion regarding the extent to which FDA oversees the compounding pharmacies that registered with FDA as drug manufacturers. Although drug manufacturers are required to register with FDA by providing company information such as name, location, and the drugs the company manufactures, compounding pharmacies meeting the FDCA's registration exemption are not required to register. However, according to FDA officials, neither the law nor the agency precludes those compounding pharmacies that are exempt from registration from voluntarily doing so, and some compounding pharmacies have registered with FDA as manufacturers and marketed themselves as "FDA-registered." FDA officials told us that registering as a manufacturer does not necessarily result in the application of regulatory requirements that apply to manufacturers or in FDA inspection for compliance with these requirements. For example, a compounding pharmacy may voluntarily register with FDA; however, this registration does not by itself give FDA authority to require the pharmacy to comply with FDA's good manufacturing practices and other requirements that apply to drug manufacturers. Nonetheless, these pharmacies appear as registered manufacturers in FDA's registration database, the Drug Registration and Listing System.

When entities that compound drugs on a large scale register with FDA as manufacturers and market themselves as "FDA-registered," it may erroneously convey an endorsement by FDA. As a result, some state officials and purchasers may incorrectly assume FDA inspects the entities or has reviewed and approved their compounded drugs. Officials from one of the national pharmacy organizations told us that they recently learned that a pharmacy can be registered with FDA as a drug establishment as well as with the state as a pharmacy. They added that healthcare professionals and the public may assume that if an entity registers with FDA then that means that FDA is in some way regulating that entity. In addition, NABP officials noted that they were aware of some entities engaged in drug compounding whose drug compounding activities are not subject to state oversight because they are registered as manufacturers with FDA and the states assume FDA is overseeing these activities. Yet, if a compounding pharmacy is voluntarily registered with FDA, the agency would not inspect it for compliance with good manufacturing practices because it does not manufacture FDA-approved drugs.

Further, FDA lacks reliable data to make decisions to prioritize its inspection workload and other follow-up and enforcement actions.[24] Under standards for internal control in the federal government, relevant, reliable, and timely information should be available for external reporting purposes and management decision making. According to FDA officials, although the agency's FACTS database has a code for inspections of compounding facilities, some compounding pharmacies could be inspected and coded as either manufacturers of human drugs or manufacturers of veterinary drugs, and the FACTS database would not identify them as inspections of compounding pharmacies. In addition, while FDA can manually look up the results of an individual inspection, the agency does not have ready access to all of the final classification of inspections for those compounding pharmacies it can identify in its FACTS database; in these instances, FACTS does not indicate the agency's final determination whether an official action was indicated, voluntary action was indicated, or if no action was indicated from the inspection results.[25] According to FDA officials, some of the final decisions are in hard copy, and the database includes recommendations from the district office inspectors, which may differ from the final inspection classifications.[26] Without reliable, timely data on all inspections conducted and the actions required and taken following those inspections, FDA lacks ready access to key data to inform its decision making on its oversight priorities and to take appropriate action when problems are identified.

In addition, pharmacies are generally not required to report to FDA adverse events regarding compounded drugs they have produced, unlike drug manufacturers who are required to report to FDA if they become aware of adverse events associated with their products. [27] Therefore, adverse event data about compounded drugs consists of voluntary reports, and FDA officials said that the agency is only aware that an adverse event involves a compounded drug if the individual voluntarily reporting the adverse event specifies that a compounded drug was involved in the event. While FDA's adverse event data associated with compounded drugs is limited, a recent report by the Pew Charitable Trusts identified 20 pharmacy compounding errors associated with 1,022 adverse events, including 75 deaths, since 2001.[28] According to this report, contamination of sterile products was the most common compounding error, though some incidents were the result of pharmacists' and technicians' miscalculations and mistakes in filling prescriptions.

Oversight of Drug Compounders Has Been Limited, but FDA Has Recently Increased Its Efforts

Until 2013, FDA limited its inspections of compounding pharmacies to those conducted in response to complaints or adverse events, called "for cause" inspections;[29] however, the agency has recently conducted inspections of compounding pharmacies that FDA identified as known to produce "high-risk" sterile compounded drugs. From its available data, FDA identified 194 "for cause" inspections of compounding pharmacies the agency conducted from February 8, 2002, through May 11, 2012, under its pharmacy compounding assignment code for human drugs.[30] Of these 194 inspections, FDA issued 63 form 483 inspection observation reports outlining significant objectionable conditions identified during the inspections. FDA subsequently issued at least 31 warning letters to pharmacies as a result of these inspections for problems such as bacterial and fungal contamination found in sterile clean rooms and in finished product samples, improper hygiene and garbing procedures (e.g., putting on gowns, gloves, and shoe covers), failure to conduct appropriate laboratory testing on drug products, and inadequate ventilation.

However, FDA has not taken any enforcement actions against the 31 entities where the agency found problems significant enough to send warning letters, according to FDA officials. Further, we found that 19 of the 194 compounding pharmacies were registered with FDA as drug manufacturers.

While FDA policy requires that the final inspection classification (which states whether official action, voluntary action, or no action was indicated based on the inspection findings) be entered into the agency's FACTS database, FDA officials said they could not readily provide the final inspection classification for the 194 inspections of compounding pharmacies. The officials said that in some cases the database included FDA district officials' recommendations for inspection classification rather than the final inspection classification.

As a result, we could not ascertain how many of the 194 inspections of compounding pharmacies found problems that were significant enough for FDA to determine that official action was indicated.

More recently, FDA began inspecting compounding pharmacies in February 2013 that, according to the agency, were known to produce "high-risk" sterile compounded drugs.[31] These inspections were not the for-cause inspections that FDA has typically done in the past when inspecting compounding pharmacies. Rather, FDA's objective was to determine whether certain pharmacies that were known to have produced high-risk sterile drug products in the past posed a significant threat to public health from poor production practices.

According to FDA officials, the agency identified 31 compounding pharmacies to inspect using criteria that included whether a warning letter had been issued to the pharmacy in the past 10 years, whether the pharmacy compounded sterile injectable drugs, whether there were adverse drug events reported, or whether there were complaints received from the FDA district office or others.

FDA officials said they also reviewed related congressional committee reports that mentioned specific pharmacies and reviewed pharmacy websites. In summarizing these efforts, FDA reported that pharmacies meeting at least two of FDA's criteria were included in the inspections.[32]

As of April 29, 2013, FDA had issued form 483 inspection observation reports to 30 of the 31 compounding pharmacies it inspected as part of its recent inspections.[33] FDA's observations included inappropriate or inadequate, or both, clothing for sterile processing, lack of appropriate air filtration systems, insufficient microbiological testing, and other practices that create risk of contamination.

As of May 21, 2013, 7 of the 31 compounding pharmacies had voluntarily recalled some or all of their sterile compounded products as a result of observations from these recent FDA inspections. [34] For example:

- FDA sampled a compounded sterile injectable solution during one of its inspections in March 2013 and found bacteria in the product, which resulted in the compounding pharmacy immediately announcing a nationwide recall of all of its sterile compounded products, which included over 50 sterile drug products.
- Another compounding pharmacy recalled its sterile drug products that had not yet reached the expiration date listed on the product because of a lack of sterility assurance. This recall included approximately 95 dosage units of various sterile compounded drugs that the pharmacy supplied to the offices of licensed medical professionals located within its state; however, some patients that received products from those medical professionals may live in other states.

Further, according to our analysis, 10 of the 31 high-risk compounding pharmacies that FDA inspected were also registered in FDA's drug manufacturer database. Even though these compounding pharmacies were registered with FDA, agency officials said the agency does not routinely inspect these pharmacies despite their registration because registration alone does not trigger a routine inspection. Additionally, 8 of the 10 were individual facilities of two different larger compounding pharmacies, both of which had websites advertising they were FDA-registered.

States and National Organizations Have Taken Various Actions to Strengthen Oversight of Drug Compounding

The four states we reviewed—California, Connecticut, Florida, and Iowa—have each recently taken actions, such as working with national pharmacy organizations, to improve their oversight of drug compounding. In addition, national pharmacy organizations have undertaken efforts to help states oversee drug compounding. However, some states may lack the resources to provide the necessary oversight of drug compounding.

The Four States Reviewed Have Taken Actions, Including Increased Inspections, to Strengthen Oversight of Drug Compounding

All four of the states we reviewed recently took steps to potentially strengthen their oversight of drug compounding. These steps included developing an inspection program for sterile drug compounders that dispense drugs in the state, but are located outside of the state, and drafting new legislation to require the board of pharmacy to conduct on-site inspections prior to licensing a pharmacy. Examples of actions taken by each of the four states we reviewed follow:

California: On May 29, 2013, the California Senate passed legislation that would prohibit any pharmacy from compounding or dispensing, and any nonresident pharmacy from compounding for shipping into the state, sterile compounded drug products unless the pharmacy has obtained a sterile compounding pharmacy license from the California Board of Pharmacy; require inspection of resident and nonresident pharmacies by the board prior to licensure; require resident and nonresident pharmacies to report adverse events for compounded drugs to both the California State Board of Pharmacy and MedWatch, FDA's adverse event reporting system; and require resident and nonresident pharmacies to submit a list of all sterile medications compounded by the pharmacy during the prior 12 months before obtaining an annual renewal of the sterile compounding license, among other requirements. Currently, California law requires that a pharmacy that compounds sterile injectable drug products in California, or that ships sterile injectable products into California, obtain a special license issued by the board; however, the law exempts from this licensure requirement certain pharmacies that have current accreditation from a private accreditation agency approved by the board.[35] California pharmacies that obtain licensure by the board are subject to prelicensure inspections, as well as annual inspections prior to renewal of the license.

Nonresident pharmacies must provide a copy of a recent inspection report issued by the pharmacy's licensing agency, or a recent report from a private accrediting agency approved by the board, documenting the pharmacy's compliance with board regulations regarding the compounding of injectable sterile drug products.

In describing the board's support of the proposed legislation, a California State Board of Pharmacy official told us that the board believed it important that all California and nonresident pharmacies compounding sterile injectable drugs be subject to state inspections, including those with an accreditation. As of June 14, 2013, the legislation was pending before a California State Assembly committee.

Connecticut: An official from Connecticut's Drug Control Division—which conducts inspections of pharmacies in the state and houses the Commission of Pharmacy Board Administrator, which oversees pharmacy licensing—told us that, as of April 2013, the state was working to tighten its regulations and implement inspection practices regarding in-state sterile drug compounders.

For example, the state plans to begin conducting more thorough pharmacy inspections in which the inspectors consider additional attributes, such as compliance with USP standards on sterile compounding, the physical environment where the facility is located, and the number of sales representatives employed by the pharmacy. In addition, the Drug Control Division is working to propose new regulations to allow the state to better track and regulate the sale of compounded sterile medications produced by resident and nonresident sterile drug compounders. However, the details of these proposed regulations were not available as of June 2013.[36]

Florida: On November 20, 2012, the Florida Board of Pharmacy issued an emergency rule requiring all resident pharmacies and nonresident pharmacies that ship drugs to Florida to immediately notify the board of their compounding activities.[37]

More than half (55 percent) of the 8,193 responding pharmacies reported that they compound nonsterile products, such as ointments or tablets; and 12 percent reported that they compound sterile products, such as injectable and ophthalmic solutions. Florida found that about one-third (32 percent) of the 946 pharmacies that perform sterile compounding were nonresident pharmacies.[38]

One goal of Florida's emergency rule was to determine the scope of sterile and nonsterile compounding within Florida's resident and nonresident licensed pharmacies.

According to Florida Board of Pharmacy officials, prior to the emergency rule, the board did not know how many pharmacies compounded drugs, how many nonresident pharmacies shipped compounded drugs into the state, or whether they compounded nonsterile or sterile drugs. According to these officials, the board intends to use this newly acquired information to improve the board's oversight activities, such as to identify and inspect compounding pharmacies.

As of May 2013, the Florida Board of Pharmacy was considering whether to require pharmacies to complete an updated survey biennially in order to renew their pharmacy licenses.

Iowa: Iowa is inspecting drug compounders that are licensed by the state as nonresident pharmacies and dispensing compounded drugs in Iowa. Iowa established a consultancy services agreement with NABP in December 2012, and inspectors from NABP began inspecting the 581 nonresident pharmacies identified by the state at that time. The results of these inspections are expected to reveal whether the selected pharmacies are compounding drugs in compliance with state regulations.

According to Iowa Board of Pharmacy officials, the state does not have information on the extent that Iowa's licensed nonresident pharmacies compound drugs, how many nonresident pharmacies ship compounded drugs into the state, or whether they compound nonsterile or sterile drugs.

However, NABP's inspections have begun to provide some of this information. As of April 2013, Iowa's Board of Pharmacy had taken six formal disciplinary actions against five out-of-state compounding pharmacies following NABP inspections and, according to an Iowa Board of Pharmacy official, the board anticipates more disciplinary actions during the remainder of 2013 and early 2014.

By the end of 2013 or early in 2014, an Iowa Board of Pharmacy official anticipates that NABP inspectors would visit all nonresident pharmacies licensed by the state.

States May Leverage National Organizations' Efforts to Enhance Oversight of Drug Compounding

At the national level, pharmacy organizations have undertaken a number of efforts to help states oversee drug compounding. For example, national pharmacy organizations have developed standards for compounded drugs that could be adopted by states.

The following are examples of efforts undertaken by national pharmacy organizations.

The National Association of Boards of Pharmacy (NABP): NABP has initiated the Compounding Action Plan to identify and inspect compounding pharmacies. It includes continued collaboration on the Iowa nonresident inspection program, discussed above, and the sharing of inspection results and related actions.

Through this plan, NABP intends to collect data on the number of compounding pharmacies, including their scope of operations, in all states, and inspect these pharmacies. NABP officials said they believe that many of the 581 nonresident pharmacies licensed and identified by the Iowa Board of Pharmacy also hold licenses with many, if not all, of the other states requiring nonresident licensure.

Using the Iowa nonresident licensed pharmacy list as a starting point, NABP sent Iowa's list to each state to confirm information regarding these pharmacies, such as whether the pharmacy has been disciplined, whether it is engaged in sterile compounding, or whether it is engaged in "nontraditional" compounding activities.

In addition, NABP asked all states to identify any known or suspected compounding pharmacies in their state that are not on the Iowa nonresident pharmacy list. As a result, NABP officials told us that NABP added some additional pharmacies to Iowa's original inspection list. As of June 2013, NABP had inspected 215 pharmacies.[39] In addition to its Compounding Action Plan, NABP created and continues to maintain a Model State Pharmacy Act and Model Rules for states to use when developing new pharmacy laws and regulations, including rules specific to sterile compounding. According to NABP officials, each state has adopted aspects of NABP's model act and model rules.[40]

The Pharmacy Compounding Accreditation Board (PCAB): In 2006, eight national pharmacy organizations established the PCAB, a voluntary accrediting organization for sterile and nonsterile drug compounders.[41] According to an organization official, PCAB's national standards are based on the consensus of industry experts of those elements that should exist in a pharmacy that adheres to high quality standards. PCAB accreditation indicates that the staff involved in compounding have proper and ongoing training; that the pharmacy uses active pharmaceutical ingredients and inactive materials from appropriate suppliers; that all compounding procedures are fully documented and carried out in conformance with established formulas; and USP standards for compounding.

According to a PCAB official, as of June 26, 2013, 176 drug compounding pharmacies received PCAB accreditation, and 124 additional drug compounding pharmacies have applied for PCAB accreditation.[42]

Resource Constraints and Other Factors May Affect States' Ability to Oversee Drug Compounding

Some states may lack the fiscal or staff resources to provide the necessary oversight of drug compounding. A number of officials from state boards of pharmacy attending a December 2012 meeting conducted by FDA expressed confidence that their states had adequate resources to oversee drug compounders, but were concerned about resources in other states. They explained that, until recently, they depended on the states where the pharmacies were located to license and regulate those pharmacies. However, many state budgets have been cut and it is uncertain whether all states have the resources or qualified staff to inspect and otherwise appropriately oversee their licensed pharmacies.

The effect of limited state resources may reach across state lines, and it may not be correct to assume that a pharmacy licensed by another state is being regulated adequately.

In addition, differences in pharmacy inspection practices among states may affect oversight of drug compounding in other states. For example, each of the four states we reviewed require licensure or registration of nonresident pharmacies that provide pharmacy services to users in the state, and they require nonresident pharmacies applying for a license or registration to have a current license, permit, or registration issued by the regulatory authority of their home state.

The states in our review also have generally relied on the home states of the nonresident pharmacies to inspect these pharmacies on a regular basis. However, state officials and officials from national pharmacy organizations we interviewed told us that the frequency of pharmacy inspections and the qualifications of the pharmacy inspectors vary widely among states, and it is uncertain whether all nonresident pharmacies receive adequate oversight from their home states. Of the four states in our review, one required annual inspections of all pharmacies located in the state and one required annual inspections of all sterile drug compounding pharmacies located in the state, while another required routine inspections of retail pharmacies in the state once every 4 years.

In addition, three of the four states required all pharmacy inspectors to have a license to practice pharmacy in that state, while one state reported having some inspectors without pharmacist licenses.

Officials representing several national pharmacy organizations that we interviewed also expressed concerns regarding whether states have enough resources to regulate and inspect pharmacies on a timely basis. Instead, some states inspect pharmacies only in response to a problem they become aware of through a complaint or adverse drug event.

Some of these officials also expressed concern regarding FDA's resources to oversee drug compounding. For example, officials from NABP told us that both FDA and the state boards of pharmacy need more resources for the oversight of drug compounding.

Recognizing the need for additional resources to oversee drug compounders, the bill that the California legislature is considering—a bill that would require nonresident pharmacies shipping sterile compounded drugs into the state to have an on-site inspection by the California Board of Pharmacy prior to licensure—would also require those pharmacies to pay for inspection-related travel expenses.

CONCLUSION

To ensure that compounding pharmacies receive adequate oversight, it is essential to have clear roles for FDA and states regarding the regulation and oversight of drug compounding. The inconsistent federal circuit court decisions complicate FDA's ability to oversee drug compounding by requiring FDA to approach the regulation of drug compounding differently in different parts of the country.

In addition, state approaches to the oversight of pharmacies, including compounding pharmacies, vary depending upon each state's regulations and the resources each state devotes to licensing and inspecting its pharmacies. Taken together, the different regulatory approaches FDA must take and the variation in how states oversee drug compounding, create gaps in oversight, which could lead to inadequate assurance that public health is protected.

To adequately carry out the oversight of compounded drugs, FDA must have data systems in place to produce timely, reliable information on inspections, the findings of those inspections, and enforcement actions taken related to compounded drugs.

Without reliable, timely data, the agency will not have the information needed to intercede and protect Americans from unnecessary harm when problems are identified.

Recent FDA inspections of 31 entities that produce compounded drugs and the subsequent drug recalls highlight the potential risk to public health of failing to oversee these types of entities.

At the same time that FDA lacks complete information on inspections and enforcement actions taken related to compounded drugs, entities that compound drugs may register as manufacturers in the agency's registration database, and some advertise themselves as FDA-registered.

As a result, states and purchasers may incorrectly assume that FDA has approved the products and inspected the facilities for compliance with good manufacturing practices.

MATTER FOR CONGRESSIONAL CONSIDERATION

To help ensure appropriate oversight of the safety of products from the entities that prepare and distribute compounded drugs that have a high potential to adversely affect public health, Congress should consider clarifying FDA's authority to regulate entities that compound drugs.

RECOMMENDATIONS FOR EXECUTIVE ACTION

We recommend that the Secretary of Health and Human Services direct the Commissioner of the FDA to

- take steps to consistently collect reliable and timely information in FDA's existing databases on inspections and enforcement actions associated with compounded drugs, and
- clearly differentiate in FDA's database, those manufacturers of FDA-approved drugs that FDA inspects for compliance with good manufacturing practices from those entities compounding drugs that are not FDA-approved and that FDA does not routinely inspect.

AGENCY COMMENTS AND OUR EVALUATION

We provided a draft of this report to HHS, which oversees FDA, for comment. HHS provided written comments and technical comments, which we incorporated as appropriate. HHS stated that our report accurately details the limitations associated with FDA's current authority to oversee drug compounding.

HHS's comments also support the Matter for Congressional Consideration that Congress should consider clarifying FDA's authority to oversee entities that compound drugs.

HHS neither agreed nor disagreed with our recommendations. Regarding our first recommendation to direct FDA to consistently collect reliable and timely information in FDA's existing databases on inspections and enforcement actions associated with compounded drugs, HHS stated that although FDA's FACTS database can be improved to better aggregate data and to facilitate evaluation of compounding pharmacy activities, these deficiencies do not materially impact FDA's ability to protect the public from harm when problems are identified.

We understand that FDA has the ability to access the data associated with compounded drugs by searching under a company name or requesting information across FDA centers and offices; however, as our report notes, FDA lacks ready access to all of the data and lacks the ability to run queries or aggregate the data. For example, when we requested the final inspection classifications for 194 inspections of compounding pharmacies, FDA could not provide this information because, according to FDA officials, the FACTS database does not contain all of the final decisions and obtaining all of the final inspection classifications would require time-consuming manual searches of information maintained in hard copy.

As a result, we could not ascertain how many of these inspections found problems that were significant enough for FDA to determine that official action was indicated. Therefore, we continue to believe that FDA should take steps to consistently collect reliable and timely information in its databases on inspections and enforcement actions associated with compounded drugs. Doing so would provide the agency with ready access to key data to inform its decision making on its oversight priorities and allow it to take appropriate action when problems are identified.

In its comments, HHS stated that FDA will take steps to further improve its databases to ensure that inspections and actions regarding compounding going forward are coded consistently and are more readily identifiable through electronic searches, and that the final classification for inspections of drug compounders are entered into the FACTS database. These steps are consistent with our recommendation.

Regarding our second recommendation, HHS stated that FDA will consider whether it would be possible or appropriate to differentiate in its database those compounding pharmacies that register voluntarily from conventional manufacturers of FDA-approved drugs that are required to register. These conventional manufacturers are already subject to routine inspections by FDA and are required to list the FDA-approved products they manufacture.

Therefore, these entities should already be known to FDA. HHS also commented that FDA will provide information to the public about what it means—and does not mean—to voluntarily register with FDA. HHS further stated that FDA has recommended that Congress require pharmacies engaged in nontraditional compounding in the United States to register with FDA and list the drugs they are compounding, all of which is consistent with our recommendation.

Marcia Crosse
Director, Health Care

APPENDIX I: INFORMATION ON SELECTION CRITERIA FOR FOUR STATES

To identify actions planned or taken by states, we interviewed representatives of the state pharmacy regulatory bodies from four states: California, Connecticut, Florida, and Iowa. We chose these states to provide insight into how a range of states approach the oversight of drug compounding; however, the approaches and experiences of these states are not generalizable to all 50 states.

We selected these states to reflect a range of characteristics, including census region, population, number of licensed pharmacies, and variation in compounding regulations. Table 1 lists select data for each selected state.

Table 1. Characteristics Considered in Selecting Four States for Inclusion in Review of State Oversight of Compounding Pharmacies

State	Census region [a]	2010 population (in millions) [b]	Number of compliance officers/ inspectors	Number of state licensed pharmacies	Number of pharmacy license categories[c]	Anticipatory Compounding requirements [d]
California	West, Pacific	37.3	37[e]	7,352 (of which 482 are nonresident) [e]	6	May compound in advance of receipt of a patient-specific prescription based on a documented history of prescriptions for the individual patients in that patient population, but only in amounts necessary to ensure continuity of care for that patient population.
Connecticut	Northeast, New England	3.6	10 (8 inspectors and 2 supervisors) [e]	1,301 (of which 624 are nonresident) [e]	6	May compound in anticipation of prescriptions based on routine, regularly-observed prescribing patterns.
Florida	South, South Atlantic	18.8	20[f]	8,050 (of which 754 are nonresident) [f]	16	May compound in anticipation of prescriptions based on routine regularly-observed prescribing patterns.
Iowa	Midwest, West, North Central	3.0	7[f]	1,510 (of which 567 are nonresident) [f,g]	4	May compound drugs prior to receiving a valid prescription based on a history of receiving valid prescriptions generated solely within an established pharmacist/patient/ prescriber relationship.

Source: GAO analysis of U.S. Census Bureau, the National Association of Boards of Pharmacy, and state pharmacy law data.

[a]U.S. Census Bureau, Census Regions.

[b]U.S. Census Bureau, 2010 state demographic profiles.

[c]The National Association of Boards of Pharmacy 2013 Survey of Pharmacy Law.

[d]Analysis of state pharmacy laws and regulations.

[e]As of April 2013.

[f]As of May 2013.

[g]The number of licensed nonresident pharmacies varies over time as new pharmacies are licensed by the state and as licensed pharmacies go out of business or otherwise discontinue their licenses.

APPENDIX II: HISTORY OF THE FOOD AND DRUG ADMINISTRATION'S (FDA) AUTHORITY OVER DRUG COMPOUNDING AND APPROACH TO OVERSIGHT

Amendments to the Federal Food, Drug, and Cosmetic Act (FDCA) enacted in 1997, and a series of federal court decisions regarding the validity of those amendments, have resulted in several significant shifts in FDA's authority and approach to the regulation of drug compounding over the last two decades.

Differences in these court decisions have resulted in inconsistent FDA authority to oversee drug compounding, which, according to the agency, has prompted it to apply three different regulatory approaches to compounded drugs depending upon the federal court jurisdiction in which the drugs are compounded. This appendix describes these legal developments.

1992-1997: Administrative Framework Established for Drug Compounding Oversight

In 1992, FDA issued a compliance policy guide that articulated the agency's approach to applying the FDCA's new drug, adulteration, and misbranding provisions to compounded drugs.[1] FDA noted its longstanding policy of deferring to state regulation of pharmacies engaged in traditional compounding activities, but that it was issuing the compliance policy guide to identify those circumstances under which the agency believed establishments with retail pharmacy licenses were engaged in "manufacturing, distributing, and promoting unapproved new drugs" in a manner outside the traditional pharmacy practice of compounding.[2] According to the 1992 compliance policy guide, the agency might exercise its enforcement discretion to take action against such establishments for violations of the FDCA's new drug approval, adulteration, and misbranding provisions.

1997-2001: Statutory Framework Established for Drug Compounding Oversight

In 1997, Congress passed and the President signed into law the Food and Drug Administration Modernization Act of 1997 (FDAMA) that, among other things, amended the FDCA to expressly permit drug compounding under certain conditions and to exempt compounded drugs meeting these conditions from certain provisions of the FDCA. In particular, under section 503A of the FDCA, as enacted by FDAMA, compounded drugs meeting these conditions were expressly exempt from the requirement that a drug be manufactured in conformity with current good manufacturing practice; that a drug's labeling carry adequate directions for use; and that the drug is the subject of an approved new drug application.

To qualify for these exemptions, the pharmacist, physician, or pharmacy compounding the drug had to meet certain criteria, including refraining from advertising, promoting, or soliciting prescriptions for the compounding of any drug.

1999-2002: Judicial Developments in the Ninth Circuit

Shortly after FDAMA's enactment, a group of seven pharmacies challenged section 503A's advertising, promotion, and solicitation restrictions in federal district court, alleging that these restrictions violated the Free Speech Clause of the First Amendment. Agreeing with the plaintiffs, the U.S. District Court for the District of Nevada invalidated section 503A's advertising, promotion, and solicitation restrictions, severing these restrictions from the remainder of section 503A.[3]

In 2001, the U.S. Court of Appeals for the Ninth Circuit affirmed the district court's First Amendment holding; however, the Ninth Circuit took the view that Congress would not have enacted section 503A without the advertising, promotion, and solicitation provisions and, therefore, the law's advertising, promotion, and solicitation provisions were not severable. As a result, it held that section 503A, in its entirety, was invalid.[4]

In April 2002, the United States Supreme *Court in Thompson v. Western States Medical Cente*r affirmed the Ninth Circuit's ruling invalidating section 503A's advertising, promotion, and solicitation provisions.[5] Because neither the government nor the pharmacies appealed the Ninth Circuit's severability ruling, the Supreme Court declined to address the validity of the remaining nonadvertising portions of section 503A.[6]

2002: Revised Administrative Framework for Drug Compounding Oversight

One month after the Supreme Court's ruling in *Western States*, FDA revised its longstanding 1992 *Compliance Policy Guide* on pharmacy compounding to provide "immediate guidance on what types of compounding might be subject to enforcement action under current law."[7] In that guidance, FDA took the position based on the Ninth Circuit's and Supreme Court's *Western States Medical Center* decisions, that "all of section 503A is now invalid." Accordingly, the agency determined it was necessary to issue guidance outlining the factors the agency would consider in taking enforcement action against a compounding pharmacy for violations of the FDCA. In particular, the agency stated that it would continue to defer to state pharmacy authorities for "less significant" violations of the FDCA but that when a pharmacy's activities resemble those of a drug manufacturer it would consider enforcement action. The compliance policy guide provides a nonexhaustive list of such activities. The compliance policy guide reflected FDA's view that, even if a compounding pharmacy has not engaged in these activities, the drugs it compounded would be subject to all of the FDCA's requirements that apply to manufactured drugs; in the compliance policy guide FDA simply outlined those circumstances under which the agency would actually enforce these requirements against a compounding pharmacy.

2006-2008: Judicial Developments in the Fifth Circuit

Four years later, in 2006, a group of 10 pharmacies challenged FDA's authority to regulate compounded drugs. In that case, FDA asserted that compounded drugs fall within the FDCA's definition of "new drug" and, therefore, are subject to those provisions of the act that apply to such drugs.[8] The U.S. District Court for the Western District of Texas disagreed with the agency, holding that compounded drugs when created for an individual patient pursuant to a prescription from a licensed practitioner "are implicitly exempt" from the FDCA's new drug definition and the new drug approval process.[9] On appeal, the U.S. Court of Appeals for the Fifth Circuit reversed the district court's determination and held that compounded drugs are "new drugs" under the FDCA.[10] The court reasoned that Congress would not have enacted FDAMA's provisions exempting compounded drugs from certain of the FDCA's "new drug" requirements had these provisions not applied to compounded drugs in the first instance.[11] To reach this conclusion, the Fifth Circuit considered the severability of section 503A's nonadvertising provisions.[12] Disagreeing with the Ninth Circuit's *Western States* reasoning that Congress would not have enacted section 503A without the advertising provisions, the Fifth Circuit found that the FDCA contained a severability provision and that this provision applied to section 503A. Finding no strong evidence that Congress would not have enacted section 503A without the advertising provisions, the court ruled that the law's nonadvertising provisions were severable from its unconstitutional provisions.[13] The result of the Fifth Circuit's decision is that—at least in the Fifth Circuit—compounded drugs are, in fact, "new drugs" under the FDCA; however, these drugs are expressly exempt from certain requirements that apply to "new drugs"—namely, compliance with current good manufacturing practice, certain labeling requirements, and new drug approval requirements—if they comply with the nonadvertising conditions set forth in section 503A.[14]

2008-Present: FDA's Different Oversight Approaches Following a Circuit Split

The Ninth Circuit Court of Appeals' 2001 *Western States* decision invalidating all of section 503A and the Fifth Circuit Court of Appeals' 2008 *Medical Center Pharmacy* decision holding that all of section 503A other than the advertising, promotion, and solicitation restrictions is valid are directly at odds. As a result of these decisions, section 503A is invalid in those states in the Ninth Circuit (Alaska, Arizona, California, Hawaii, Idaho, Montana, Nevada, Oregon, and Washington) and in full force and effect in those states in the Fifth Circuit (Louisiana, Mississippi, and Texas). FDA officials described the agency's approach to regulating compounded drugs under this incongruous legal landscape as follows:

- In the Ninth Circuit, the agency takes the approach that all compounded drugs are "new drugs" under the FDCA, and the agency determines whether to consider taking enforcement action against a compounding pharmacy based on whether the pharmacy engages in any of the activities outlined in the agency's 2002 compliance policy guide on drug compounding. Even if a compounding pharmacy has not engaged in the activities outlined in the compliance policy guide, the drugs it compounds are, as a legal matter, subject to all of the

FDCA requirements that apply to "new drugs"; the compliance policy guide simply outlines those circumstances under which the agency will consider enforcing these requirements against a compounding pharmacy.[15]

- In the Fifth Circuit, FDA determines whether a compounded drug meets section 503A's exemption from certain FDCA requirements that would preclude the agency from taking enforcement action against a drug compounder for noncompliance with these requirements.
- For compounding pharmacies outside of the Fifth and Ninth Circuits, which is the majority of the country, the agency applies the criteria in both section 503A and its 2002 compliance policy guide to determine whether to take enforcement action.

Table 2 identifies the criteria that a compounded drug must meet to qualify for the exemption under section 503A of the FDCA from certain of the law's requirements and the criteria in FDA's 2002 compliance policy guide, which the agency considers in determining whether to take enforcement action against an entity engaged in drug compounding.

Table 2. Comparison of the Food and Drug Administration's (FDA) Authority and Oversight of Drug Compounding under Section 503A of the Federal Food, Drug, and Cosmetic Act (FDCA) and FDA's 2002 Compliance Policy Guide

Section 503A: A drug compounded according to each of the criteria isexempt from three key requirements under the FDCA. [a]	2002 Compliance Policy Guide:In determining whether to initiate enforcement actionagainst a compounding pharmacy, FDA considers whetherthe compounding pharmacy has engaged in any of theseactivities. [b,c,d]
Compounds for an identified individual patient based on the receipt of a valid prescription order or a notation, approved by the prescribing practitioner, on the prescription order that a compounded drug is necessary for the patient. If compounding occurs in anticipation of a prescription, it is based on a history of valid prescription orders for the compounding of the drug	Compounding in anticipation of receiving prescriptions, except in very limited quantities in relation to the amounts of drugs compounded after receiving valid prescriptions.

Section 503A: A drug compounded according to each of the criteria isexempt from three key requirements under the FDCA. [a]	**2002 Compliance Policy Guide:In determining whether to initiate enforcement actionagainst a compounding pharmacy, FDA considers whetherthe compounding pharmacy has engaged in any of theseactivities.** [b,c,d]
product, which orders have been generated solely within an established relationship between the pharmacy and the prescriber or patient.	
Does not compound a drug product that appears on a list published by the Secretary of drug products withdrawn or removed from the market because such drug product or their components have been found to be unsafe or not effective	Compounding drugs withdrawn or removed from the market for safety reasons
Compounds using ingredients (other than bulk drug substances) that comply with an applicable monograph	Receiving, storing, or using drug components not meeting official compendia requirements
Compounds using bulk drug substances that comply with an applicable compendia monograph if one exists; if one does not exist, uses bulk drug substances that are components of FDA-approved drugs or that appear on a list developed by the agency e	Compounding finished drugs from certain bulk active ingredients that are not components of FDA approved drugs without an investigational new drug application
Compounds with bulk drug substances that were made in an FDA-registered facility, each of which is accompanied by valid certificates of analysis	Receiving, storing, or using drugs substances without obtaining assurance they were made in an FDA-registered facility
Compounds in a state that has entered into a memorandum of understanding with the Secretary that addresses the distribution of inordinate amounts of compounded drug products interstate and provides for appropriate investigation by a state agency of complaints relating to compounded drug products distributed outside of the state; in the alternative, less than 5 percent of the compounding individual's or entity's total prescription orders are for compounded products distributed out of the state	Compounding drugs for third parties who resell to individual patients or at wholesale to other persons or entities or using commercial scale manufacturing or testing equipment for compounding drug products

Table 2. (Continued)

Section 503A: A drug compounded according to each of the criteria isexempt from three key requirements under the FDCA. [a]	**2002 Compliance Policy Guide:In determining whether to initiate enforcement actionagainst a compounding pharmacy, FDA considers whetherthe compounding pharmacy has engaged in any of theseactivities.** [b,c,d]
Does not compound regularly or in inordinate amounts (as defined by the Secretary) any drug products that are essentially copies of a commercially-available drug product f	Compounding drugs that are commercially available or that are essentially copies of commercially-available FDA-approved drug products, except in certain limited circumstances.
Does not compound any drug that is identified by the Secretary by regulation as a drug that presents demonstrable difficulties for compounding that reasonably demonstrate an adverse effect on the safety or effectiveness of that drug	*No comparable criterion*
The compounding is performed by a licensed pharmacist in a state licensed pharmacy or by a licensed physician.	Failing to operate in conformance with applicable state pharmacy laws

Source: GAO analysis.

Notes: Data are from section 503A of the Federal Food, Drug, and Cosmetic Act and FDA's 2002 compliance policy guide on drug compounding.

Section 503A's advertising, promotion, and solicitation restrictions are not presented here, as the United States Supreme Court declared these provisions unconstitutional. *Thompson v. W. States Med. Ctr.*, 535 U.S. 357 (2002).

[a]FDA applies these criteria to drugs compounded in states other than those in the Ninth Circuit, where section 503A is invalid, to determine whether these drugs are exempt from certain FDCA requirements.

[b]FDA applies these criteria in states outside of the Fifth Circuit to determine whether to initiate enforcement action against a compounding pharmacy in such a state.

[c]For compounding pharmacies outside of the Fifth and Ninth Circuits, FDA applies the criteria in both section 503A and the 2002 compliance policy guide to determine whether to take enforcement action.

[d]In addition to the specific factors outlined in the 2002 compliance policy guide, according to FDA, the agency also considers whether a licensed practitioner has extemporaneously compounded a drug upon receipt of a valid prescription for an individually identified patient in considering whether to take enforcement action.

[e]FDA issued a proposed rule on January 7, 1999, containing a list of bulk drug substances that the agency proposed to permit for use in drug compounding. 64

Fed. Reg. 996 (Jan. 7, 1999). According to FDA, the agency never issued a final rule because of the Ninth Circuit's and Supreme Court's *Western States* decisions. Since the Fifth Circuit Court of Appeals' 2008 *Medical Center Pharmacy* decision, the agency has considered whether to maintain such a list.

[f]The term "essentially a copy of a commercially-available drug product" does not include a drug product in which there is a change, made for an identified individual patient, which produces for that patient a significant difference, as determined by the prescribing practitioner, between the compounded drug and the comparable commercially available drug product.

End Notes

[1] While drug compounding is often referred to as "pharmacy compounding," physicians may compound drugs in certain instances. The focus of this review is drug compounding by pharmacies.

[2] FDA is responsible for assuring the safety and effectiveness of these drugs regardless of whether they are manufactured in the United States or abroad.

[3] 21 U.S.C. §§ 301 *et seq.*

[4] The contaminated product was traced to a compounding pharmacy in Massachusetts, which had shipped approximately 17,000 vials of a contaminated injectable steroid to 23 states. According to the Centers for Disease Control and Prevention, as of July 1, 2013, 749 individuals who received the contaminated steroid injections became ill with fungal meningitis or other types of infections, and 61 of them have died.

[5] See GAO, *Prescription Drugs: State and Federal Oversight of Drug Compounding by Pharmacies,* GAO-04-195T (Washington, D.C.: Oct. 23, 2003).

[6] We selected four states based on variations in geography, population, organization of pharmacy regulatory bodies, and pharmacy compounding laws and regulations.

[7] NABP is a professional association that assists its member state boards of pharmacy and jurisdictions in developing, implementing, and enforcing uniform standards for the purpose of protecting the public health. USP is a scientific nonprofit organization that sets standards for the identity, strength, quality, and purity of medicines, food ingredients, and dietary supplements. For this report, we refer to these organizations, including those representing pharmacies and pharmacists, as national pharmacy organizations.

[8] These standards provide an overall framework for establishing and maintaining internal controls; and for identifying and addressing major performance and management challenges, and areas at greatest risk of fraud, waste, abuse, and mismanagement. See GAO, *Standards for Internal Control in the Federal Government*, GAO/AIMD-00-21.3.1 (Washington, D.C.: November 1999), and its supplemental guide, *Internal Control Management and Evaluation Tool*, GAO-01-1008G (Washington, D.C.: August 2001).

[9] GAO-04-195T.

[10] Department of Health and Human Services, Office of Inspector General, *High-Risk Compounded Sterile Preparations and Outsourcing by Hospitals That Use Them* (Washington, D.C.: Apr. 10, 2013).

[11] USP's current suite of General Chapters for compounding includes: Chapter 797 Pharmaceutical Compounding—Sterile Preparations, which provides procedures and

requirements for compounding sterile preparations; Chapter 795 Pharmaceutical Compounding—Nonsterile Preparations, which provides guidance on applying good compounding practices in the preparation of nonsterile compounded formulations for dispensing and/or administration to humans or animals; Chapter 1160—Pharmaceutical Calculations in Prescription Compounding; Chapter 1163—Quality Assurance in Pharmaceutical Compounding; and Chapter 1176—Prescription Balances and Volumetric Apparatus. According to USP officials, these compounding chapters reference an additional 48 USP chapters. In addition to setting standards that affect compounding, USP, through the *United States Pharmacopeia-National Formulary*, a compendium of public pharmacopeial standards, provides monographs for drug articles, including ingredients used in compounded preparations, and monographs for the compounded preparations themselves, comprising standards of identity, quality, purity, strength, packaging, and labeling.

[12] National Association of Boards of Pharmacy, *Survey of Pharmacy Law—2013* (Mount Prospect, IL: 2013). The pharmacy regulatory bodies of Guam and Puerto Rico also reported that they require compliance with USP's standards on sterile compounding.

[13] The FDCA defines "new drug" as "Any drug ... the composition of which is such that such drug is not generally recognized, among experts qualified by scientific training and experience to evaluate the safety and effectiveness of drugs, as safe and effective for use under the conditions prescribed, recommended, or suggested in the labeling thereof. . . . ." 21 U.S.C. § 321(p)(1). Drug manufacturers submit new drug applications to FDA to seek approval to market and sell a new pharmaceutical drug product in the United States. In addition, abbreviated new drug applications are submitted to FDA to seek approval to market a generic version of a drug after the period of exclusivity and any patents for a brand-name drug expire. In fiscal year 2013, user fees for new drug applications ranged from $979,400 to $1,958,800, depending on whether or not the application required clinical data, and were $51,520 for abbreviated new drug applications.

[14] Pub. L. No. 105-115, § 127, 111 Stat. 2296, 2328 (Nov. 21, 1997). Compounded drug products that met these requirements did not have to comply with good manufacturing practices, label drugs with adequate directions for use, or have an FDA-approved new drug or abbreviated new drug application. References to section 503A in this report are to section 503A of the FDCA, as codified at 21 U.S.C. § 353a.

[15] A pharmacy's records are exempt from FDA's inspection authority if the pharmacy is in compliance with any applicable local laws regulating the practice of pharmacy and medicine, regularly engages in dispensing drugs upon a prescription from a licensed practitioner, and does not manufacture, prepare, or compound drugs for sale other than during the regular course of its business of dispensing or selling drugs at retail. 21 U.S.C. § 374(a)(2)(A).

[16] An FDA form 483 is an inspection observation report that lists objectionable conditions observed at the facilities. An FDA warning letter is a correspondence that notifies a responsible individual or firm that the agency considers one or more products, practices, processes, or other activities to be in violation of the FDCA, its implementing regulations, and other federal statutes.

[17] 21 U.S.C. § 360.

[18] A pharmacy is exempt from these registration and listing requirements if the pharmacy is in compliance with any applicable local laws regulating the practice of pharmacy and medicine, regularly engages in dispensing drugs upon a prescription from a licensed practitioner, and does not manufacture, prepare, or compound drugs for sale other than

during the regular course of its business of dispensing or selling drugs at retail. 21 U.S.C. § 360(g)(1).

[19]According to FDA officials, the agency typically seeks inspection warrants when inspection has been refused completely or when refusals have been encountered in limited areas (e.g., when a firm has refused to allow FDA to take photographs or collect samples). FDA officials also reported having to obtain warrants to inspect 2 of 31 compounding pharmacies it inspected in 2013.

[20]21 U.S.C. § 374(a)(2)(A).

[21] For example, Statement of Janet Woodcock, M.D., Director, Center for Drug Evaluation and Research, FDA, before the Senate Committee on Health, Education, Labor, and Pensions, 113th Cong., May 9, 2013.

[22] On June 19, 2013, the Senate Committee on Health, Education, Labor and Pensions reported out of committee a bill that would create a new category of "compounding manufacturer," which is similar in some respects to FDA's proposed category of "nontraditional drug compounder." Pharmaceutical Compounding Quality and Accountability Act, S. 959, 113th Cong. (1st Sess. 2013). In addition, on May 23, 2013, a bill was introduced in the House of Representatives, H.R. 2186, to strengthen federal oversight of drug compounding. VALID Compounding Act, H.R. 2186, 113th Cong. (1st. Sess. 2013).

[23] Pharmacies are not required to register with FDA if they follow any applicable local laws regulating the practice of pharmacy and medicine, regularly engage in dispensing drugs upon a prescription from a licensed practitioner, and do not manufacture, prepare, or compound drugs for sale other than during the regular course of their business of dispensing or selling drugs at retail. 21 U.S.C. § 360(g)(1).

[24] We have previously reported on weaknesses in the data FDA uses to prioritize its inspection workload, including FACTS. See, for example, GAO, *Drug Safety: Better Data Management and More Inspections Are Needed to Strengthen FDA's Foreign Drug Inspection Program*, GAO-08-970 (Washington, D.C.: Sept. 22, 2008).

[25] FDA classifies an inspection as "official action indicated" if objectionable conditions were found that warrant regulatory action by the agency. A classification of "voluntary action indicated" means that objectionable conditions were identified but any corrective actions are left to the establishment to take voluntarily. A classification of "no action indicated" means that no objectionable conditions or practices were found during the inspection (i.e., conditions or practices that violate current good manufacturing practices), or if the significance of the documented objectionable conditions found does not justify further FDA action.

[26] According to FDA officials, the agency does not have ready access to all of the final inspection classifications as some of the records are in hard copy and it would be difficult and time consuming to review the inspection reports and any associated documentation to evaluate and determine why certain final decisions were made or not made. Agency officials told us that reasons why a final decision was not entered into its FACTS database include, but are not limited to, the difficulty of the agency to come to a final classification determination on an inspection due to the complexity of legal issues associated with the regulation of compounded drugs and compounding pharmacies or failure to enter the data.

[27] Generally, if a manufacturer receives drug- or certain device-related adverse event reports, it must send them to FDA. Health care professionals and consumers can voluntarily file adverse event reports with FDA and may also report these events to the products' manufacturers. User facilities (e.g., hospitals and nursing homes) must report certain

device-related—but not drug-related—adverse events to FDA as well. 21 C.F.R. §§ 314.80(c), 803.30, 803.50.

[28] The Pew Charitable Trusts is an independent, nonprofit research and public policy organization. Pew Charitable Trusts, American Society of Health-System Pharmacists, American Hospital Association, *Pharmacy Sterile Compounding Summit: Summary of a Stakeholder Meeting* (Washington D.C.: Apr. 15, 2013).

[29] FDA's inspection plan for fiscal year 2011 called for five full-time equivalent staff to inspect compounding pharmacies, and its plan for fiscal year 2012 called for two full-time equivalent investigator staff for these inspections.

[30] FDA officials noted that this is likely an incomplete list of inspections of compounding pharmacies. That is, they said that the agency could have conducted additional inspections of compounding pharmacies; but they could only identify 194 of them because of limitations in FDA's inspections database. According to FDA officials, additional inspections may have been coded as investigations rather than inspections (although they involved inspectional activity as part of the investigation) and some inspections of compounding pharmacies could have been coded as inspections of human drug manufacturers.

[31] For FDA's summary describing these inspections, see Food and Drug Administration, *Summary: 2013 FDA Pharmacy Inspection Assignment*, accessed April 30, 2013, http://www.fda.gov/Drugs/GuidanceComplianceRegulatoryInformation/PharmacyCompounding/ucm347722.htm. FDA officials told us that to conduct these inspections of compounding pharmacies the agency had to take inspectors off other assignments.

[32] According to FDA officials, the agency used a risk-based model to identify the pharmacies and 15 of the 31 pharmacies had at least one reported death and, thus, were included in FDA's inspections regardless of whether they met any of the other criteria.

[33] According to FDA officials, 1 of the 31 pharmacies the agency inspected did not receive an FDA form 483, and this pharmacy was not compounding sterile drugs. Four of the 31 pharmacies were individual facilities of one pharmacy firm, and 4 others were individual facilities of another firm; however, FDA counted each facility as a separate compounding pharmacy.

[34] In addition, as of May 30, 2013, four other compounding pharmacies that were not part of the 31 pharmacies inspected by FDA initiated voluntary recalls of their sterile compounded products because of concerns of a lack of sterility assurance. FDA identified bacterial and fungal growth in samples of a sterile compounded drug in a subsequent inspection of one of these compounding pharmacies.

[35] Resident pharmacies operated by entities that are licensed by either the board or the California Department of Health and nonresident pharmacies operated by entities that are licensed as a hospital, home health agency, or a skilled nursing facility are eligible for such exemption. Cal. Bus. & Prof. Code §§ 4127.1, 4127.2. In contrast to current law, which imposes special licensure requirements only on pharmacies compounding injectable sterile drugs, the proposed legislation would require pharmacies compounding all types of sterile drugs to meet such requirements.

[36] In Connecticut, pharmacy licensure and pharmacy inspections are handled separately. The state's Commission of Pharmacy, which is administered by the Department of Consumer Protection, is responsible for approval of new licenses. The commission also adjudicates cases involving pharmacists, pharmacies, and pharmacy technicians brought before it. The Department of Consumer Protection's Licensing Division handles the clerical aspects of licensing pharmacists and pharmacies while the state's Department of Consumer Protection,

Drug Control Division, conducts pharmacy inspections and implements enforcement actions. Connecticut has 10 drug control agents who conduct pharmacy inspections, all of whom are licensed pharmacists.

[37] Specifically, Florida's emergency rule required resident pharmacies with state pharmacy permits and nonresident pharmacies registered with the state to immediately notify the board of their sterile and nonsterile compounding activities, the types of drugs they compound, and whether they compound drugs in bulk. In addition, the emergency rule required Florida's board of pharmacy to use the information on compounding activities to place a high priority on inspecting high-risk pharmacies such as those that compound sterile drugs. The emergency rule also required all nonresident registered pharmacies to provide a copy of their last two inspection reports as provided by the state in which the pharmacies are physically located and licensed.

[38] Florida Department of Health, Division of Medical Quality Assurance, *Florida Board of Pharmacy Compounding Survey Report* (Tallahassee, FL: Jan. 23, 2013).

[39] NABP will also assist the New Jersey Division of Consumer Affairs with inspections of New Jersey pharmacies engaged in the practice of compounding under a recently reached agreement with the New Jersey Division of Consumer Affairs and the state's Attorney General. New Jersey licenses approximately 40 retail pharmacies that perform sterile compounding and 109 hospital pharmacies that may compound sterile products. NABP inspectors will assist the division in performing field inspections at compounding pharmacies, detailed audits of their records, and in-depth analysis of inspection findings. In addition, NABP inspectors will assist with investigations into complaints about compounding pharmacies, and in bringing charges against any found to be noncompliant.

[40] NABP's Model State Pharmacy Act and Model Rules (Model Act) provide state boards of pharmacy with model language that may be used when developing state laws or board rules. The Model Act includes sections on the boards of pharmacy, licensing (pharmacists, technicians, and facilities), and discipline. NABP last updated the Model State Pharmacy Act and Model Rules in August 2012.

[41] The following national pharmacy organizations established PCAB and, with the exception of the National Association of Boards of Pharmacy, currently make up PCAB's Board of Directors: American College of Apothecaries, National Community Pharmacists Association, American Pharmacists Association, National Alliance of State Pharmacy Associations, International Academy of Compounding Pharmacists, National Home Infusion Association, National Association of Boards of Pharmacy, and the United States Pharmacopeial Convention.

[42] According to a PCAB official, as of June 24, 2013, 176 PCAB-accredited pharmacies were located in 41 states and no state or other entity required PCAB accreditation for a pharmacy to compound drugs.

End Notes for Appendix II

[1] FDA, Compliance Policy Guides, § 460.200 Manufacture, Distribution, and Promotion of Adulterated, Misbranded, or Unapproved New Drugs for Human Use by State-Licensed Pharmacies (Mar. 16, 1992).

[2] The compliance policy guide describes such traditional compounding to include compounding of "reasonable quantities of drugs upon receipt of a valid prescription for an individually identified patient from a licensed practitioner."

[3] *W. States Med. Ctr. v. Shalala*, 69 F. Supp. 2d 1288 (D. Nev. Sept. 16, 1999).

[4] *W. States Med. Ctr. v. Shalala*, 238 F.3d 1090 (9th Cir. Feb. 6, 2001).

[5] *Thompson v. W. States Med. Ctr.*, 535 U.S. 357 (2002).

[6] *Id.* at 360.

[7] FDA, Compliance Policy Guide § 460.200 Pharmacy Compounding (May 29, 2002).

[8] Section 201(p) of the FDCA defines "new drug" as "Any drug ... the composition of which is such that such drug is not generally recognized, among experts qualified by scientific training and experience to evaluate the safety and effectiveness of drugs, as safe and effective for use under the conditions prescribed, recommended, or suggested in the labeling thereof." 21 U.S.C. § 321(p).

[9] *Med. Ctr. Pharmacy v. Gonzales*, 451 F. Supp. 2d 854, 863, 865 (D.W.D. Tex. Aug. 30, 2006).

[10] The Fifth Circuit vacated the district court's judgment and remanded the case to the district court for further proceedings. *Med. Ctr. Pharmacy v. Mukasey*, 536 F.3d 383, 409 (5th Cir. Jul. 18, 2008).

[11] *Id.* at 400 ("In 1997, Congress enacted FDAMA as an amendment to the FDCA. That amendment provides considerable evidence that Congress sought to address pharmacy compounding directly and that it did so with the assumption that the 'new drug' provision applies to drugs created through pharmacy compounding.")

[12] *Id.* at 401 ("[T]o rely on FDAMA in construing the 'new drug' definition, we first must address FDAMA's validity.").

[13] *Id.* at 402, 404-05.

[14] *Id.* at 405.

[15] The Ninth Circuit Court of Appeals decision also applies to FDA's authority over certain compounding pharmacies located in Colorado, New Jersey, Tennessee, Texas, and Wisconsin, as these pharmacies were party to the *Western States* lawsuit.

In: Drug Compounding
Editor: Martti Bram
ISBN: 978-1-63117-360-8

Chapter 4

STATEMENT OF JANET WOODCOCK, DIRECTOR, CENTER FOR DRUG EVALUATION AND RESEARCH, FOOD AND DRUG ADMINISTRATION. HEARING ON "EXAMINING DRUG COMPOUNDING"*

INTRODUCTION

Mr. Chairman and Members of the Subcommittee, I am Dr. Janet Woodcock, Director of the Center for Drug Evaluation and Research at the Food and Drug Administration (FDA or the Agency), which is part of the Department of Health and Human Services (HHS). Thank you for the opportunity to be here today to discuss important issues related to pharmacy compounding.

We are at a critical point where we must work together to improve the safety of drugs produced by compounding pharmacies. As the compounding industry has grown and changed, we have seen too many injuries and deaths over many years caused by unsafe practices. Dr. Margaret Hamburg, Commissioner of Food and Drugs, testified in front of the Oversight and Investigations Subcommittee on April 16, 2013, regarding the emergence of a tragic fungal meningitis outbreak associated with compounded methylprednisolone acetate (MPA), a steroid injectable product distributed by

* This is an edited, reformatted and augmented version of a presentation on May 23, 2013 before the House Energy and Commerce Committee, Subcommittee on Health.

the New England Compounding Center (NECC). To date, that outbreak has been associated with 55 deaths and over 740 people sickened in 20 States. Sadly, NECC was not an isolated incident. Indeed, over the past 20 years we have seen multiple situations where compounded products have caused deaths and serious injuries. For example:

- In 1997, two patients were hospitalized with serious infections after administration of contaminated riboflavin injection prepared by a Colorado pharmacy.
- In 2001, 13 patients in California were hospitalized and 22 received medical care following injections from contaminated vials of a steroid solution. Three patients died as a result.
- In 2002, five patients in North Carolina suffered from fungal meningitis resulting from contaminated methylprednisolone acetate made by a South Carolina pharmacy. One person died.
- In 2005, contaminated cardioplegia solution, made by a firm located in Maryland, resulted in five cases of severe system inflammatory infections; three of these patients died.
- In 2007, three people died from multiple organ failure after a Texas compounder sold superpotent colchicine that was as much as 640 percent the labeled strength.
- In 2010, FDA investigated a cluster of *Streptococcus endophthalmitis* bacterial eye infections in patients who received injections of Avastin repackaged by a pharmacy in Tennessee.
- In 2011, there were 19 cases of *Serratia marcescens* bacterial infections, including nine deaths, associated with contaminated total parenteral nutrition products.
- In 2012, 43 patients developed fungal eye infections from contaminated sterile ophthalmic drug products. At least 29 of these patients suffered vision loss.
- Recently, in 2013, FDA investigated reports of five cases of eye infections in patients who received Avastin repackaged by a pharmacy in Georgia. The Avastin was contaminated with bacteria.

These incidents are emblematic of long-standing issues associated with the practice of compounding and the public health concerns that can result from unsafe practices in compounding pharmacies.

Since the NECC outbreak, ten additional firms have conducted voluntary recalls overseen by FDA of sterile compounded or repackaged drug products as of May 16, 2013. In one recent incident, the presence of floating particles, later identified to be a fungus, was reported in five bags of magnesium sulfate intravenous solution, resulting in a nationwide recall of all sterile drug products produced by the pharmacy (over 100 products). Fortunately, we have not received reports of patient injury from these products. In another recent recall, all sterile drug products (approximately 60 products) from a second pharmacy were recalled as a result of reports that five patients were diagnosed with serious eye infections associated with the use of repackaged Avastin. Moreover, we believe that presently, there are hundreds of other firms operating as compounding pharmacies, producing what should be sterile products and shipping across State lines in advance of or without a prescription. However, the current legal framework does not provide FDA with the tools needed to identify and appropriately regulate these pharmacies to prevent product contamination.

The history of this issue shows that there is a need for appropriate and effective oversight of this evolving industry. It is clear that the industry and the health care system have evolved and outgrown the law, and FDA's ability to take action against compounding that exceeds the bounds of traditional pharmacy compounding and poses risks to patients has been hampered by limitations and ambiguities in the law, which have led to legal challenges to FDA's authority to inspect pharmacies and take appropriate enforcement actions.

The fungal meningitis outbreak has caused the Agency to review our past practices with regard to our oversight of compounding pharmacies, and has led to some preliminary conclusions. In my view, even in the face of litigation and continuous challenges by industry to our authorities, we can nonetheless be more aggressive in pursuing enforcement actions against compounding pharmacies within our current authority. I can assure you that we are being more aggressive now. We have established an Agency-wide steering committee to oversee and coordinate our efforts, and we have taken several important steps to identify and inspect high-risk pharmacies that are known to have engaged in production of sterile drug products.

Using a risk-based model, we identified 29 firms for priority inspections focused on their sterile processing practices. During these 29 inspections, in two instances, FDA identified secondary firms associated with the priority inspections, for a total of 31 firms. We have taken investigators who would normally be doing inspections of conventional drug manufacturers and assigned them to conduct inspections of those pharmacies whose history suggests a greater risk of potential quality issues with their compounded products. We have coordinated our inspections with State officials, who have accompanied our investigators in most cases. At the same time, we have also continued to conduct for-cause inspections, often at the request of our State counterparts who invited us to accompany them on the inspections. Since the fall, FDA has completed 26 for-cause inspections in addition to the 31 described above, as of May 16, 2013. When we identified problems during any of the inspections, at the close of the inspection, we issued an FDA Form 483[1] listing our inspection observations. We have issued an FDA-483 at the close of 47 of the 57 inspections we have conducted since last fall. We have seen some serious issues, including quality concerns that have led to product recalls. Observations have included: lack of appropriate air filtration systems, insufficient microbiological testing, and other practices that create risk of contamination.

Notably, even in light of recent events, and even though we are often working with the State inspectors, our investigators' efforts are being delayed because they are denied full access to records at some of the facilities they are inspecting. Just during the recent inspections, several pharmacies delayed or refused FDA access to records, and FDA had to seek administrative warrants in two cases. And although we have been able to eventually conduct the inspections and collect the records that we have sought, our ability to take effective regulatory action to obtain lasting corrective action with regard to substandard sterility practices remains to be seen.

As we have noted in the past, our ability to take action against inappropriate compounding practices has been hampered by ambiguities regarding FDA's enforcement authority, legal challenges, and adverse court decisions, and we have learned that the law is not well-suited to effectively regulate this evolving industry. For example, hospitals have come to rely on compounding pharmacies that function as "outsourcers" producing sterile drugs previously made by hospital in-house pharmacies. If FDA brings charges against a pharmacy, alleging that it is manufacturing a "new drug" that cannot be marketed without an approved application, the pharmacy will have to either obtain individual patient-specific prescriptions for all of its products or stop distributing the products until it obtains approved new drug applications for them, something most outsourcers are unlikely to do. Several of the pharmacies FDA inspected are some of the largest outsourcers in the country. These pharmacies supply large numbers of sterile drugs produced in relatively large quantities to hospitals nationwide, and a shut-down at these firms is likely to cause disruptions in the supply of drugs to hospitals and other health care providers. FDA should have more tailored authorities appropriate for this type of compounding pharmacy.

In the Commissioner's appearances before the Committee on Energy and Commerce in November 2012 and April 2013, she presented a framework that could serve as a basis for the development of a risk-based program to better protect the public health, improve accountability, and provide more appropriate and stronger tools for overseeing this evolving industry. Since November, we have met with over 50 stakeholder groups, including pharmacy, medical, hospital, payer, and consumer groups, and State regulators, to help further our understanding and inform our framework. Today, I will first provide background on FDA's current legal authority over compounded drugs, then review that framework, and suggest specific actions that Congress can take to help us better do our job and prevent future tragedies like this one.

FDA's Legal Authority over Compounded Drugs

FDA regards traditional pharmacy compounding as the combining or altering of ingredients by a licensed pharmacist, in response to a licensed practitioner's prescription for an individual patient, which produces a medication tailored to that patient's special medical needs. In its simplest form, traditional compounding may involve reformulating a drug, for example, by removing a dye or preservative in response to a patient allergy. It may also involve making an alternative dosage form such as a suspension or suppository for a child or elderly patient who has difficulty swallowing a tablet. FDA believes that pharmacists engaging in traditional compounding provide a valuable medical service that is an important component of our health care system. However, by the early 1990s, some pharmacies had begun producing drugs beyond what had historically been done within traditional compounding.

After receiving reports of adverse events associated with compounded medications, FDA became concerned about the lack of a policy statement on what constituted appropriate pharmacy compounding. In March 1992, the Agency issued a Compliance Policy Guide (CPG), section 7132.16 (later renumbered as 460.200) to delineate FDA's enforcement policy on pharmacy compounding. It described certain factors that the Agency would consider in its regulatory approach to pharmacies that were producing drugs.

The compounding industry objected to this approach and several bills were introduced, some with significant support, to limit the Agency's oversight of compounding.[2] In November 1997, S. 830, the Food and Drug Administration Modernization Act of 1997 (FDAMA), was signed into law as Public Law 105-115.[3] FDAMA added Section 503A to the FD&C Act, to address FDA's authority over compounded drugs.[4] Section 503A exempts compounded drugs from three critical provisions of the FD&C Act: the premarket approval requirement for "new drugs"; the requirement that a drug be made in compliance with current good manufacturing practice (cGMP) standards; and the requirement that the drug bear adequate directions for use, provided certain conditions are met. These provisions were the subject of subsequent court challenges, which have produced conflicting case law and amplified the perceived limitations and ambiguity associated with FDA's enforcement authority over compounding pharmacies. In 2002, immediately after a Supreme Court ruling that invalidated the advertising provisions of Section 503A, FDA issued a revised compliance policy guide on compounding human drugs. Several additional legal challenges and court decisions then followed. More recently, FDA made significant progress toward issuing another CPG. In fact, FDA was on track to publish a revised draft CPG in the fall of 2012, but the fungal meningitis outbreak intervened and we are now reevaluating the draft. It is important to note, however, that a CPG is not binding on industry and updating the CPG would not alleviate all issues with Section 503A. A look at FDA's attempts to address compounding over the last 20 years shows numerous approaches that were derailed by constant challenges to the law. As a result, presently, it is unclear where in the country Section 503A is in effect, and Section 503A itself includes several provisions that have impeded FDA's ability to effectively regulate pharmacy compounding practices including those relating to prescription orders, medical need, and copying FDA-approved products.

Apart from Section 503A, there are additional provisions in the statute that have impeded effective pharmacy compounding regulation. For example, if certain criteria are met, the FD&C Act exempts compounding pharmacies from registration and the obligation to permit access to records during an inspection. As a result, FDA has limited knowledge of pharmacy compounders and compounding practices and limited ability to oversee their activities.

Looking Ahead

The Administration is committed to working with Congress to address the threat to public health from limitations in authorities for effective oversight of certain compounding practices. To that end, FDA has developed a framework that could serve as the basis for the development of a risk-based program to protect the public health.

Risk-Based Framework

Recognizing the history of compounding practice, FDA supports the long-standing policy that all compounding should be performed in a licensed pharmacy by a licensed pharmacist (or a licensed physician), and that there must be a medical need for the compounded drug.

Further, we believe there should be a distinction between two categories of compounding: traditional and non-traditional. Traditional compounding would include the combining, mixing, or altering of ingredients to create a customized medication for an individual patient with an individualized medical need for the compounded product, in response to a valid patient-specific prescription or order from a licensed practitioner documenting such medical need. Traditional compounding, while posing some risk, plays an important role in the health care system, and should remain the subject of State regulation of the practice of pharmacy.

Non-traditional compounding would include certain types of compounding for which there is a medical need, but that pose higher risks. FDA proposes working with Congress to define nontraditional compounding based on factors that make the product higher risk such as any sterile compounding in advance of or without receiving a prescription, where the drug is distributed out of the state in which it was produced. Non-traditional compounding would be subject to Federal standards adequate to ensure that the compounding could be performed without putting patients at undue risk, and FDA would inspect against and enforce these Federal standards. Such a definition focuses on the highest risk activities and offers a uniform degree of protection across all 50 States, for highest-risk compounding activities.

Non-traditional compounding should, because of the higher risk presented, be subject to a greater degree of oversight. Sterile products produced in advance of or without a prescription and shipped interstate should be subject to the highest level of controls, established by FDA and appropriate to the activity, similar to cGMP standards applicable to conventional drug manufacturers.

In addition, FDA believes that with noted exceptions, certain products are not appropriate for compounding under any circumstances. These products would include: 1) what are essentially copies of FDA-approved drugs, absent a shortage justification based on the drug appearing on FDA's shortage list; and 2) complex dosage forms such as extended release products; transdermal patches; liposomal products; most biologics; and other products as designated by FDA. Producing complex dosage forms would require an approved application and compliance with cGMP standards, along with other requirements applicable to manufactured drug products.

FDA believes that there are other authorities that would be important to support this new regulatory paradigm. For example, FDA should have clear ability to collect and test samples of compounded drugs and to examine and collect records in a compounding pharmacy, just as the Agency does when inspecting other manufacturers. FDA should also have clear ability to examine records such as records of prescriptions received, products shipped, volume of operations, and operational records such as batch records, product quality test results, and stability testing results. Such inspections are necessary to determine when a pharmacy exceeds the bounds of traditional compounding, to respond to public health threats, and to enforce Federal standards.

FDA also believes that an accurate inventory of pharmacies engaged in non-traditional compounding would facilitate appropriate oversight and coordination with State regulators. In addition, FDA looks forward to working with the Congress on potential improvements that may include label statements and adverse event reporting that have proven useful in other areas. A user-fee-funded regulatory program may be appropriate to support the inspections and other oversight activities outlined in this framework. We look forward to working with Congress to explore the appropriate funding mechanisms to support this work, which could include registration or other fees, as Congress has authorized and FDA has successfully implemented in other settings.

CONCLUSION

Given our experiences over the past 20 years and the recent fungal meningitis outbreak, we must do everything we can to clarify and strengthen FDA's authority in this area.

I am happy to answer any questions you may have.

End Notes

[1] A form FDA-483 is issued when investigators observe any significant objectionable conditions. It does not constitute a final Agency determination of whether any condition is in violation of the Federal Food, Drug, and Cosmetic Act (FD&C Act) or any of our relevant regulations, but the observations often serve as evidence of a violation of the FD&C Act and its implementing regulations.

[2] H.R. 5256, Pharmacy Compounding Preservation Act of 1994, introduced Oct. 7, 1994, 1 co-sponsor; H.R. 598, Pharmacy Compounding Preservation Act of 1994, introduced Jan. 20, 1995, 141 co-sponsors; H.R. 3199, Drug and Biological Products Reform Act of 1996, introduced March 29, 1996, 205 co-sponsors; H.R. 1060, Pharmacy Compounding Act, introduced March 13, 1997, 152 co-sponsors; H.R. 1411, Drug and Biological Products Modernization Act of 1997, introduced April 23, 1997, 16 co-sponsors

[3] Public Law 105-115, FDAMA, 111 Stat. 2296 (Nov. 21, 1997), available at http://www.gpo.gov/fdsys/pkg/PLAW105publ115/pdf/PLAW-105publ115.pdf

[4] Id.

In: Drug Compounding
Editor: Martti Bram
ISBN: 978-1-63117-360-8

Chapter 5

TESTIMONY OF SCOTT GOTTLIEB, RESIDENT FELLOW, THE AMERICAN ENTERPRISE INSTITUTE. HEARING ON "EXAMINING DRUG COMPOUNDING"*

KEY POINTS

1. There exists a practice of pharmacy. It was never intended that all compounding would create a new drug and be subject to Food and Drug Administration regulation but for the enforcement discretion of the FDA or for the willingness of Congress to provide explicit exemption to certain pharmacists and certain activities.
2. FDA has authority to target compounders that cross the line between the practice of pharmacy and engage in drug manufacturing under the guise of a pharmacy license. While legal precedents cited by other witnesses have created some ambiguity, what the FDA largely lacks is ease of administering its authority. FDA is generally not able to force firms to submit advance information to FDA (before the firm is suspected of any wrongdoing) so that the agency is able to more efficiently identify firms engaged in wrongdoing and target its oversight. In some cases, FDA doesn't know about these firms until a problem arises. In other instances, FDA is forced to make an affirmative case that a compounding pharmacy is violating the law

* This is an edited, reformatted and augmented version of a presentation on May 23, 2013 before the House Energy and Commerce Committee, Subcommittee on Health.

before the agency is able to compel an inspection or take other measures.

3. FDA generally lacks tools and/or resources to regulate a new class of firms that the agency has dubbed "non traditional compounders". I would argue that the firms in question here are not compounders, and calling them such confuses different issues. These are firms that repackage sterile FDA approved products into new dosage forms to improve their administration and enable the drugs to be tailored to therapy – for example, breaking chemotherapy into pediatric volumes, mixing hyperalimentation, preparing IV fluids, and breaking hospital-volume anesthetics like propofol for use in appropriately supervised outpatient settings. These firms fall into a gray area right now where they are treated as compounders but are not engaging in traditional forms of compounding. Rather they are engaging in the bulk repacking and manufacturing sterile preparations of FDA approved drugs, in advance of (and often not in response to) prescriptions for individual patients. To the degree that these large-scale operations prepare sterile volumes of drugs in a bulk form and ship these units widely, they present some novel risks.
4. As we address issues of supply, we also must address the policy decisions that have increased demand for compounded products from large scale "non traditional" compounders. At times, FDA has exercised its authority unevenly, which has given more incentive to compounders to skirt the law. Also FDA's actions against generic firms have driven the market for many drugs to compounders. In law and regulation, we need to take a risk-based approach that encourages sourcing of drugs from the most competent parts of the market, not its least competent elements.
5. This is going to be especially important if we create a new class of compounders that FDA has dubbed "non traditional compounding". If FDA doesn't exercise its authority evenly, which means not allowing firms to compound identical versions of FDA approved products, then FDA will give incentive for drug makers to re-mask themselves as "non traditional compounders" to skirt the new drug requirements.
6. Part of the reason why FDA's oversight has been, at times, inconsistent is that the agency often had a product orientation -- not a facility-based orientation – to its enforcement activity. That needs to change. FDA often targeted products they believed were being inappropriately marketed for inappropriate uses, rather than firms that

were not operating under sound conditions. Enforcement was often reactive as a result. The agency's enforcement needs to take on both considerations.

7. Finally, the market for compounded drugs is evolving quickly. It's consolidating, and other entities (distributors, generic manufacturers) could well start buying out the large compounders. To these ends, what we do today may be irrelevant to the market we see in the near future. It may pay to wait and see how things shake out, and also to see how FDA's recent enforcement activity impacts these markets.

The views expressed in this testimony are those of the author alone and do not necessarily represent those of the American Enterprise Institute.

INTRODUCTION

Mr. Chairman Pitts, Mr. Ranking Member Pallone, and members of the House Energy and Commerce Committee, Subcommittee on Health:

Thank you for the opportunity to testify today before this Committee.

The tragic deaths of 55 Americans and sickening of more than 740[1], resulting from contaminated steroid injections (methylprednisolone acetate) that were shipped by a disreputable "compounding pharmacy" located in Massachusetts, have rightly focused public attention and the work of this Committee on a largely unfamiliar, but prominent part of our drug supply chain – the practice of pharmacy compounding.

Before this House Committee, as well as the Senate, are proposals to tighten federal regulatory oversight of these compounding pharmacies, and of the practice of pharmacy more generally. Observers are calling on Congress to give the Food and Drug Administration (FDA) expanded oversight of these establishments.

New laws merit consideration. We should articulate clear and bright lines between the legitimate practice of pharmacy compounding, and those firms operating illegally as large-scale drug manufacturers under the guise of a pharmacy license.

I don't believe that it should be left to FDA's discretion to establish these boundaries as the agency goes about its work, or allow a fuzzy standard to persist. I believe that this would only add to uncertainty in the marketplace and create an undue burden on FDA to interpret vague authority. Ultimately it would result in uneven enforcement that would risk repeating some of the past mistakes.

Nor do I believe any pharmacy practice where drugs are compounded necessarily creates a new drug. There is such a thing as the practice of pharmacy that was, in my view, a sphere of medical practice that was never intended to be subject to FDA oversight. There are pharmacies that clearly practice within the scope of their profession, and are subject to state and professional regulation. And there are pharmacy compounders that are clearly crossing the line between the practices of pharmacy and taking on all the characteristics of a drug manufacturers and, as such, already fall squarely within FDA's existing oversight and authority.

But it seems illogical, inconsistent with prior statute, and administratively burdensome to declare that all pharmacy compounding – even done locally, for individual patients, and in response to valid prescriptions – creates a new drug and could be subject to FDA oversight but for Congress' willingness to exempt certain activity from new drug requirements, or FDA's exercise of enforcement discretion.

Instead, we should establish a clear boundary and objective tests for when pharmacies are engaging in legitimate compounding – and are subject to state regulation; and when establishments have crossed the line and are operating as drug manufacturers under the facade of a pharmacy license. When these lines are crossed, FDA has clear authority to assert – at the least – its Good Manufacturing (GMPc) standards to ensure the safety and effectiveness of products. This basic principle exists today, and should be part of any further clarification of existing law.

The merit in considering these issues is made urgent by the tragedy in Massachusetts and the apparent malfeasance at the New England Compounding Center (NECC). But it's also made necessary by the changing face of this industry.

These changes in the way compounding pharmacies operate, along with policy decisions (some made by FDA) that have increased demand for these compounded products, have strained FDA's existing resources and its policies in this area.

These challenges may call for a greater role for both state and federal regulators. But we need to be mindful of the reasons why the practice of pharmacy has traditionally been left to state regulation. When proper oversight demands that regulators examine the relationship between a provider and a patient (as proper oversight of the practice of pharmacy entails) then these endeavors are best left to state and professional authorities who have more proximity to the actual provision of care. Not every regulatory endeavor benefits from federal involvement.

In addition, we also need to be mindful of the policy decisions that drive more widespread – and sometimes inappropriate – use of compounded products. Finally, we need to be aware of the authority that FDA currently has that – with proper attention and perhaps additional resources – could provide better protections.

We need to take measure of these things before we enact new laws.

The recent problems didn't arise from traditional compounding, which is a legitimate part of the practice of pharmacy and an important part of medical care.

The traditional practice of pharmacy compounding is generally regarded as the combining or altering of ingredients by a licensed pharmacist, in response to a licensed practitioner's prescription for an individual patient. This activity produces a medication tailored to a patient's special medical needs. Compounding pharmacies mix or alter drug ingredients to adapt a medicine based on a doctor's prescription— for example by changing a pill into a formula, changing dosage forms, tailoring chemotherapy, or adding cherry flavoring to a child's medicine.

The practice of pharmacy compounding lets physicians customize drugs to individual patients. Traditional pharmacy compounding typically is performed on a small scale and is always performed in response to a valid patient prescription.

The FDA normally doesn't get involved with such practices because it isn't tasked with regulating the legitimate practice of pharmacy. Like the practice of medicine, pharmacy is largely left to professional and state oversight. But once pharmacies begin manufacturing and shipping medicines on a wide scale, and do so in a way that isn't in response to a valid prescription, these firms often become "drug manufacturers" and fall squarely under the FDA's extensive authority.[2]

In recent years, we have seen much more widespread use of compounded pharmacy products. Along with this increased use, we have seen the simultaneous expansion in the scope of the industry, and the advent of very large compounding pharmacies that commercialize and distribute drugs on a wide scale, without a doctors' prompting, and outside the boundaries of an individual patient encounter.

These mega establishments stretch the traditional definition of what it means to be a compounding pharmacy. It's the intersection between the activities of these nontraditional establishments and existing state and federal regulation, that I believe bears closer scrutiny. With my testimony today I want to do three things:

First, I want to outline some policy decisions that I believe have increased demand and weakened oversight of compounding under FDA's existing authorities.

I believe these policy decisions merit scrutiny, and perhaps re-examination. The compounding industry has evolved significantly in recent years, in many cases magnifying old risks and creating new ones. Some of this evolution owes to changes in the market for these products. But in other cases, it stems from changes in regulation that have shifted the market away from traditional manufactures, and at times, emboldened compounders to expand production into gray areas.

All of these factors bear close scrutiny. Any solution to mitigate existing risks must address not only the supply of higher-risk products, but also the factors that create the demand for these products to be produced by lower-standard manufactures.

Moreover, if Congress does seek to give FDA clearer authority to regulate these so-called non-traditional compounders, who I believe already fall outside the traditional practice of pharmacy and are subject to FDA oversight today, there is an important consideration. This new authority has to go hand-in-hand with vigorous enforcement by FDA of rules that prohibit compounders from making copies of FDA-approved drugs. Otherwise, creating this third category of "compounding manufacturers" where the full brunt of FDA's requirements don't apply will create incentive for drug manufacturers to re-cast themselves as non-traditional compounders so that they can float into this new, regulatory-light category.

In recent years, FDA has been reluctant to stop compounders from copying FDA-approved drugs out of economic concerns that it would limit consumers to higher priced products. These economic concerns have to be addressed separately.

If the NDA process imposes costs that end up raising the price of finished goods, that has to be separately addressed, perhaps through thoughtful review of how the NDA process could be made more efficient when it comes to certain lower risk, better understood sterile products. But so long as FDA is going to create a new category of compounding manufactures, it needs to prevent traditional FDA approved products from moving into this new category and undermining the safety of products now being produced by reputable manufacturers to high standards. We also need to make sure that the intellectual property surrounding those NDA products is not deliberately undermined by a new category of FDA-sanctioned manufacturers.

Second, I want to outline where FDA has existing authority to regulate nontraditional pharmacy compounding, and try and give this committee a sense for how, in my view, that authority has been exercised by FDA and why the agency has made certain choices in how it interpreted those rules. Much is made of FDA's concern that legal challenges to the existing statute and policies have left FDA's current authority muddled. While these complaints have merit, I believe that there are other considerations that also shape the strength of FDA's authority.

For example, FDA often targets specific products rather than troubled facilities. The FDA has also, at times, not enforced rules evenly out of concern that knocking certain violating products and firms out of the market might impose higher costs on consumers. All of these considerations and policy choices have merit. But they create a regulatory scheme that is at times reactive and can appear arbitrary.

Third and finally, I want to propose some ideas for how I believe that a clearer standard in policy and law could provide for more effective oversight in this area and create a clearer boundary between the legitimate practice of pharmacy compounding and those firms that are distorting that traditional custom.

FDA has noted that legal challenges to its existing policies have served to muddle its authority. We also need to consider the way that FDA's own actions have contributed to this haziness. The FDA's influence on stoking some of the challenges it now faces is instructive because as I will explain, it speaks to the need for FDA and Congress, to establish a clear line between the activities that fall within the FDA's scope and those that are traditional pharmacy left to state authority.

The Evolution of Large Scale Compounding

As FDA Commissioner Dr. Peggy Hamburg stated in recent testimony, the practice of pharmacy compounding has undergone an evolution in recent decades. We have seen the advent of very large scale compounding firms that operate with many of the characteristics of traditional drug manufacturers. In recent months, FDA has referred to this practice as "non traditional compounding."[3]

Part of this growth in compounding has been driven by greater sourcing of these products by hospitals. As Dr. Hamburg stated in recent testimony, to save costs, hospitals have outsourced compounding that they used to do in house.[4]

Let me elaborate on this point. While I agree with the FDA's general analysis, I would cast the different pieces of this broader industry into different slices.

What have evolved are essentially three types of outfits when it comes to the area generally referred to as compounding.

First is traditionally compounding, where a pharmacy works in consultation with a physician to tailor a product based on a valid prescription.

This practice of pharmacy falls within professional and state purview and has not been the source of recent concerns.

Next, there are firms that masquerade as pharmacies, but engage in large scale manufacturing, often of unique products or drugs designed to compete with FDA approved medicines. These firms develop these drugs in bulk, without valid prescriptions or in anticipation of prescriptions, and do not adhere to good, sterile manufacturing techniques. These firms seem to be violating current federal law. Many are manufacturing new and unapproved drugs. In so doing, they are already subject to FDA's current and extensive oversight.

There is a third category of manufacturers that FDA has dubbed "non traditional compounding" but which I would offer is not compounding in its traditionally form, but another new and vital manufacturing service that has evolved over time.

Firms in this third category typically produce sterile products in bulk, usually to supply large medical practices and hospitals. In its most common form, these outfits will break down large volumes of FDA approved products into smaller units, for example taking large units of an anesthetic and breaking it into syringes to be more easily administered, taking a large unit chemotherapeutic and breaking it into smaller units to be dosed for a pediatric indication, or producing hyperalimentation for supplemental nutrition delivered by parental or enteral means.

These outfits are really sterile repackaging and re-mixing firms – not compounders in the traditional, local sense. Hospitals used to do this sort compounding of work in house, in their own pharmacies. When it was a hospital-based pharmacist working on a small scale under a sterile hood, there was manageable risk and a lower likelihood of wide contamination. But to save costs and improve quality and efficiency (in part, as a response to the tightening of the hospital industry's regulations) the hospitals have outsourced this work to these new, large firms.

The firms now performing this role are doing it on a wide scale, and are not compounders in the traditional sense. FDA confuses the issues by referring to these firms as "non traditional compounders". I would call these firms sterile preparation manufacturers or sterile prep manufacturers. These firms are a new, and important category of drug suppliers. They are now a vital part of the drug supply chain for hospitals and large outpatient practices. And their work creates certain risks.

If generic drug firms were engaging in this activity, FDA would require separate drug applications for each dosage firm. FDA would require the generic firms to do stability studies, container closure studies, and pay separate user fees, among other things. This is one of the reasons why the generic drug makers do not supply drugs in the full range of dosage forms and packaging – and why the hospitals have to turn to these "sterile prep manufacturers" (or non-traditional compounders).

This begs the question: Should these sterile prep manufacturers be subject to the same oversight as a generic drug firm engaging in the same activity?

It's a relevant question, but I think the answer is no. Because these hospital preps and repackaged drugs have a shorter dating period, it might be reasonable to subject them to a lighter regulatory touch.

The firms doing this sort of "non traditional compounding" (to borrow FDA's poorly suited lexicon) generally do a good job. But they have been the source of some problems, including some fatal contaminations in recent years. A review of FDA's recent oversight work has found that these products are not uniformly produced under sterile techniques, and in some cases have some significant contaminations. To the degree these "sterile" products are being used in hospitalized patients, who often have a lot of co-morbid illness, this can create public health risks.

It is reasonable to consider whether these outfits should be subject to GMP requirements to make sure they adhere to sterile techniques.

I would offer that these firms should be the focus of the present discussion.

Traditionally compounding should continue to be the domain of state and professional oversight. And the compounders like NECC engaged in manufacturing new drugs already fall under FDA's current scrutiny. As for the sterile prep manufacturers (or "non traditional compounders") since the sterile preps and repackaged goods are often produced and shipped on a wide scale, an inadvertent contamination in one lot could have widely distributed risks before a product could be recalled by an overlapping patchwork of state and federal authority.

Policy Choices and the Rising Demand for Compounded Products

To exam why the industry has grown and evolved in recent years, also requires a closer examination of the policy measures that I believe have contributed to these circumstances. Some of these recent policy decisions have driven demand away from traditional manufacturers like generic drug firms, and to compounders.

In at least some cases, providers are turning to a small number of unreliable compounders because they cannot sources these products elsewhere.

To begin, a recent tightening in FDA's oversight of generic drug firms that made nearly identical versions of the same sterile injectable drugs produced by many compounders (including NECC) has prompted providers to source more products from large scale compounders. This tightening was rooted in some legitimate concerns that FDA had about the reliability of the generic manufacturing facilities. But it has created a contradictory set of policies that at has had the effect of shifting purchases from more reliable sources to firms with more questionable practices.

A key question is this: Even assuming that the FDA's concerns around the generic drug makers were all proven correct, would the continued production of drugs from these facilities – under close FDA supervision – been preferable to the alternative outcome -- closing these generic facilities and driving some providers to source products that were in shortage from compounders. By driving the generic firms to close their facilities while they underwent remediation, it left the market to be supplied by the only outfits still capable of operating – the compounders. This fueled further growth of these compounded products. But one must also ask whether the overall risk to the public was increased as a result of the fact that so much of the utilization had shifted to these more lightly regulated outfits.

This question is important is because it gets to the heart of the kinds of considerations that a risk-based approach to regulating these products should take up, and to how we make sure clinical needs are met with the most reliable products available. This same challenge has played out in other contexts where the decisions that FDA took may have served to increase demand for compounded drugs.

For example, Congress intended for FDA's enforcement over compounding to take into consideration when drugs were being manufactured by compounders that competed directly with FDA approved medicines, and therefore didn't offer any unique tailoring or differentiation that was a key clinical characteristic of the practice of pharmacy and the traditional role of compounding.

To these ends, the FDA has historically asserted its authority when compounding pharmacies were supplying their own versions of drugs that were also available commercially -- as FDA-approved branded and generic products. In these circumstances, the FDA held that these compounding firms were guilty of distributing unapproved new drugs. Among other things the New England Compounding Center, the outfit behind the tainted steroid shots, was cited for this sort of activity in that 2006 warning letter that FDA sent to the troubled firm.

However, a policy change made in recent years curtailed some of the exercise of this authority. This policy change gave greater economic incentive and political license to compounders to engage in more widespread production of drugs that exist as FDA approved products and compete directly with FDA regulated medicines.

In particular, FDA changed a longstanding guidance document that stipulated that the agency would clear the market of compounded drugs once a drug went through the new drug approval process and earned FDA approval for the same indication.

The guidance was changed to read that FDA would use its discretion in such cases, and only take action to remove the compounded products in cases where it had specific public health concerns. While I understand the agency's economic concerns around the potential for drug costs to rise when compounders are forced to exit the market, these considerations should not factor into the consistency by which the agency applies its policy. There are other avenues to address these economic concerns. FDA could also give greater consideration to the cost of the NDA process and ways to make that more efficient, especially in the case of old, well-understood drugs seeking FDA approval to sell approved versions of compounded drugs.

But the policy of removing the older, unapproved drugs remains controversial, and expectations that FDA would enforce it were largely squashed after FDA said it would not step in when the company KV Pharma, sought and received FDA's nod for Makena, an approved form of a type of progesterone that's widely compounded.

The FDA decided not to take action out of a well-publicized concern about the high cost of Makena relative to the compounded formulations. This political decision undermines the incentive for other companies to run registration trials to get FDA approval for drugs that are widely compounded. It emboldened compounders. The company that got FDA approval for Makena, KV Pharma, went into bankruptcy.

What kind of incentive does that give to other firms to invest in the development of FDA-approved versions of drugs that are being widely compounded?

The intervention in the KV Pharma case sends a message to would-be violators that the pricing of products could factor into how the FDA can enforce its own safety rules. The New England Compounding Center was also among the compounding firms distributing an unapproved version of the KV Pharma product. Does this committee believe that it's a good outcome that the active ingredient in Makena is now being widely used in woman who are pregnant, and made by firms like NECC?

Or would an FDA approved version of that medicine be preferable?

It's hard to have it both ways when it comes to these matters. That's why it was important that FDA lay out clear lines and enforces them vigorously and consistently to reduce the incentive of firms to skirt the law by operating as new drug manufacturers under the guise of a pharmacy license.

This is especially true if Congress creates a third category of "non traditional compounders". If FDA doesn't vigorously and consistently enforce a clear boundary between drugs that must be compounded because of the way they are made, and those that have gone through the NDA process and exist in the market as FDA approved new drugs, then the agency will create a clear and improper incentive for some drug manufacturers to re-cast themselves as "non traditional compounders" to skirt the new drug requirements of the Act. Congress should be aware that there are significant, competing tradeoffs as a result of this approach. For example, there's the potential for new policies to drive compounders out of certain popular markets.

The Exercise of FDA's Existing Authorities

Even while we consider new legislation, we should first look for avenues to help FDA make better use of its existing authority to regulate non-traditional pharmacy compounding. As FDA has shown with its recent, robust actions, the agency has some clear authority in this space and the ability to exert considerable oversight.

Indeed, by FDA's account, it targeted 29 firms for inspections based on their sterile processing practices and took stern actions against some of those firms. In most cases FDA was able to exercise its oversight without interference. In a few instances FDA needed to seek a court's backing to get access to the records. While this may have imposed some brief delays, the agency seems to have fulfilled its mission.

Much is made of FDA's concern that legal challenges to the existing statute and to the agency's policies have left FDA's current authority muddled.

While these complaints have some merit, I believe there are other considerations that also shape the exercise of FDA's authority. Considering these can provide a fuller understanding of the challenges that FDA faces, and potential policy solutions.

In particular, I believe that the FDA has historically taken a product approach to its enforcement of its compounding oversight, rather than a facility based approach. What I mean by this, more specifically, is that the enforcement actions were often taken in response to individual products that the FDA was concerned with – either because the products carried inappropriate claims, or were being used for circumstances where FDA didn't believe that the benefits justified the risks.

For example, in 2006 FDA sent a series of warning letters to compounders who were formulating topical lidocaine for use as a pre-treatment in electrolysis, to help numb peoples' legs before they had the sometimes-painful procedure.

FDA was rightly concerned that using large amounts of topical lidocaine in this way could cause systemic side effects, and was an inappropriate use of the drug.

I use this example to illustrate a simple point: That the enforcement activity often targeted the products rather than the facilities. This often made the agency's enforcement a reactive process, rather than a pro-active assessment of risk. While products being used in inappropriate ways create risks, and deserve regulatory scrutiny, the FDA can probably get as much, if not more bang for its public health dollar by bringing equal or even greater focus on the facilities that are inappropriately compounding products in ways that are unsterile and cross the line between traditional compounding and the wholesale manufacture of new drugs.

It's a difference of where the enforcement mindset emanates from – whether it flows from the drug reviewers in charge of reviewing products, or facility inspectors in charge of overseeing the quality of facilities, or some combination of each.

In the past, a lot of the enforcement activity emanated from the drug review divisions and the drug center's office of compliance. This let to an orientation that sometimes targeted products, rather than facilities. FDA would bring enforcement actions in cases where FDA found drugs that were being compounded for uses that the agency believed created risk, or misled consumers.

I believe an equal focus should be placed on targeting unsafe, unsanitary facilities whose business practices violate existing law. This requires a greater role for the FDA field in doing actual inspectional work that focuses on unsafe facilities as much as it requires a focus by drug review staff on the products themselves, and the indications they are used for.

Establishing Bright Regulatory Lines

Above all else, the inspectional activities must be targeted in a way that creates a clear delineation between the protected practice of pharmacy, and those firms that are creating new, unapproved drugs, or the sterile prep manufacturers I spoke of.

FDA has outlined a number of key factors that establish the boundary between traditional and "non traditional" compounding pharmacy. So it has historically articulated where a boundary could rest. These principles should guide policy.

It's these factors that have been the basis of FDA's recent vigorous and successful oversight efforts in this area. The agency's recent enforcement work demonstrates that the agency is able to enforce its supervision when firms fall outside of these boundaries. Moreover, some of these factors have already formed the basis of Congressional statute in section 503(A). These factors should form one basis of FDA's enforcement going forward and any re-articulation of that policy.

It's noteworthy that size, as well as shipping across state lines, alone, are not reliable criteria. There are good reasons why some products may be produced on a large scale even in response to physician prescriptions. For example, it may not be possible to develop a single dose from a bulk ingredient.

So a pharmacy producing a drug for a single physician in response to a single prescription may be forced to produce extra volumes of the same finished product.

There are equally good reasons why some pharmacies might ship products interstate. It could be as simple as a pharmacy that resides close to a state border. Proper criteria involve more than just one or several factors, but a multi-part test.

FDA has expressed some of the factors that would be part of a multi-part test in its prior guidance documents that addressed its enforcement. They include:

1. Compounding of drugs in anticipation of receiving prescriptions, except in very limited quantities that are done in close relation to the amounts of drugs that will need to be compounded after receiving valid prescriptions.
2. Compounding drugs that were already withdrawn by FDA or removed from the market for safety reasons.
3. Compounding finished drugs from bulk active ingredients that are not components of FDA approved drugs without an FDA sanctioned investigational new drug application (IND) in accordance with 21 U.S.C. § 355(i) and 21 CFR 312.
4. Receiving, storing, or using drug substances (for use in compounding) without first obtaining written assurance from the supplier that each lot of the drug substance has been made in an FDA-registered facility.
5. Receiving, storing, or using drug components not guaranteed or otherwise determined to meet official compendia requirements.
6. Using commercial scale manufacturing or testing equipment for compounding drug products.
7. Compounding drugs for third parties who resell to individual patients or offering compounded drug products at wholesale to other state licensed persons or commercial entities for resale.
8. Except in certain narrow circumstances, compounding drug products that are commercially available in the marketplace or that are essentially copies of commercially available FDA-approved drug products.
9. Failing to operate in conformance with applicable state law regulating the practice of pharmacy.

CONCLUSION

FDA has rightly noted that non-traditional compounding should, because of the higher risk presented, be subject to a greater degree of oversight. The large scale compounding we've seen in the marketplace, where firms manufacture large volumes of sterile products, and do so in advance of (and sometimes without) a proper physician prescription, and then ship these finished products across the country, should be subject to a higher level of manufacturing controls.

"Compounders" operating in this manner are not operating as pharmacies. Let's make no mistake. They are making new sterile dosage forms on a mass scale.

Other "compounding pharmacies" operating with these same characteristics, and making unapproved new drugs (like NECC) already fall outside the traditional practice of pharmacy and make themselves subject to FDA's oversight.

FDA's main complaint, in my opinion, isn't that these entities aren't subject to the agency's regulation under the existing law. The FDA's main complaint, when you boil it down, is that the existing legal framework puts too much burden on FDA (in the agency's opinion) to have to make the affirmative case that these firms are operating in a way that places them under the agency's jurisdiction. That's a valid complaint, but it' a different concern than the one commonly reported.

At its core, the issues we are talking about here aren't issues of whether or not FDA has proper authority. They do. The issues are whether or not FDA has the legal and regulatory tools to make its role in these regulatory endeavors administratively easier, more consistent and anticipatory, and less resource intensive.

FDA's traditional regulatory posture is to compel the submission of information to the agency that allows FDA to target its regulatory oversight. In the case of compounding pharmacies, FDA – at the margins – needs to often make the affirmative case that certain firms are not acting as pharmacies but as drug manufacturers and are therefore subject to the agency's oversight.

What FDA wants, in my view, is the means to compel the submission of certain information that would enable FDA to more easily demonstrate when compounders are no longer acting as compounders. But we should be candid about this key fact. Legislation could be narrowly tailored to address the real problems here. I believe that some of the proposals address issues that are peripheral to the key challenge.

In closing, I wish to make one final point. The market for compounding is changing very rapidly, not only as a result of the tragedy in Massachusetts, but the stepped up oversight that FDA has exerted in recent months, as well as the activity on Capitol Hill. It's also driven by issues in the marketplace itself, where certain lower margin businesses are looking to get into higher margin work in drug manufacturing.

To these ends, we're seeing compounders consolidate, and get acquired by more reputable manufacturers. It's my belief that this industry will undergo an evolution in the next few years, where many of the large-scale compounders will either consolidate or close because they can't meet the current scrutiny, and reputable manufacturers and maybe drug distributors will acquire many others.

We may also benefit from seeing the culmination of FDA's recent enforcement activity, and get a better sense of the contours of FDA's existing influence.

As this process unfolds, it will leave behind a much different compounding industry. This should serve as a cautionary note to all of us. The rules that we might write today may no longer be applicable to the market that we see tomorrow.

The market forces that are transforming this industry may accomplish many of the public health goals that we seek to address through legislation.

# # #

Dr. Scott Gottlieb is a physician and Resident Fellow at the American Enterprise Institute. From 2005-2007 he served as the FDA's Deputy Commissioner for Medical and Scientific Affairs, and before that as the agency's Director of Medical Policy Development and as a Senior Advisor to the FDA Commissioner. Dr. Gottlieb consults with and invests in biopharmaceutical companies and serves as a director to several life science companies. Scott Gottlieb is a member of the policy boards to the Leukemia and Lymphoma Society and the Society of Hospitalist Medicine.

End Notes

[1] CDC Statistics: http://www.cdc.gov/hai/outbreaks/meningitis.html.

[2] A compounding fracture at the FDA. Scott Gottlieb and Sheldon Bradshaw. The Wall Street Journal, November 14, 2012. A24.

[3] Pharmacy Compounding: Implications of the 2012 Meningitis Outbreak, Statement of Margaret A. Hamburg, M.D., Commissioner of Food and Drugs, Food and Drug Administration, Department of Health and Human Services, Before the Committee on Health, Education, Labor and Pensions United States Senate. November 15, 2012.

[4] Statement of Margaret A. Hamburg, MD Commissioner of Food and Drugs, Food and Drug Administration, Before the Subcommittee on Oversight and Investigations, Committee on Energy and Commerce, U.S. House of Representatives. "A Continuing Investigation Into the Fungal Meningitis Outbreak and whether it Could have Been Prevented." April 16, 2013.

In: Drug Compounding
Editor: Martti Bram

ISBN: 978-1-63117-360-8

Chapter 6

TESTIMONY OF JOE HARMINSON, OWNER OF DFW PRESCRIPTIONS, ON BEHALF OF THE NATIONAL COMMUNITY PHARMACISTS ASSOCIATION. HEARING ON "EXAMINING DRUG COMPOUNDING"*

Chairman Pitts, Vice-Chairman Burgess, Ranking Member Pallone and Members of the Subcommittee, my name is Joe Harmison and I am a pharmacist, owner of DFW Prescriptions and past president of the National Community Pharmacists Association (NCPA). NCPA appreciates the opportunity to share the community pharmacy perspective regarding issues relating to drug compounding. NCPA represents the interests of America's community pharmacists, including the owners of more than 23,000 independent community pharmacies. According to a NCPA member survey, almost 86% of independent community pharmacies compound medications. Our members perform a wide variety of compounding services including hormone replacement medications, making suspensions palatable for pediatric patients, different dosage forms for patients suffering from intractable nausea and vomiting, and medications for cystic fibrosis patients, to name a few. Specific to my practice, I compound medications primarily used in the treatment of pain that help patients and their physicians treat their conditions.

---

* This is an edited, reformatted and augmented version of a presentation on May 23, 2013 before the House Energy and Commerce Committee, Subcommittee on Health.

We are compliant with U.S. Pharmacopeial Convention (USP) <797> Pharmaceutical Compounding—Sterile Preparations standards.

Our hearts go out to the families who have suffered from the tragic event surrounding the New England Compounding Center (NECC), and NCPA is committed to working with Congress on the issue of practices that exceed state regulated compounding. NCPA commends the Committee for taking a closer look at what actions and inactions led to the tragic NECC event. We believe the Committee is taking the proper steps to address this tragedy by focusing on investigations into what steps should have been taken and oversight to ensure that the appropriate regulatory bodies are exercising their full authority.

Importance of Access to Compounded Medications

Compounding is a backbone of pharmacy practice and for many decades independent community pharmacists have provided millions of adults, children, and animals with access to safe, effective and affordable medications through compounding services. When manufactured drugs aren't an option, independent community pharmacists provide traditional pharmacy compounding to prepare customized medications for patients in accordance with a prescription based on the patient's individual needs. Compounding services can help bridge the gaps during times of prescription drug shortages. Drug shortages have nearly tripled, according to the FDA, and their impact can be devastating. Patients must be assured that they are not forced to go without needed medications or treatments because their medication is unavailable and compounding of that medication is prohibited or tied up in bureaucracy.

It is important to reiterate that pharmacist compounding is an integral part of the pharmacy profession and meets patients' needs in hospitals, long-term care and assisted living facilities, home infusion settings, and many community settings.

State Board of Pharmacy Oversight of Pharmacy Compounding Is Critical

NCPA has always and will continue to advocate that pharmacy compounding is best regulated by the state Boards of Pharmacy while manufacturing is overseen by the FDA. Pharmacy compounding of medications is an important part of medical care that allows for the dispensing of custom-made medications and should continue to be regulated by state Boards of Pharmacy, as all other medical licensed professional practices are. These state Boards of Pharmacy currently oversee all aspects of a pharmacy from licensure, oversight of pharmacists and technicians, the process of filling prescriptions, records, documents, and compliance with the state's laws and regulations. If the FDA has a concern about an appropriately-licensed pharmacy, then the FDA currently has the authority to ask the state Board of Pharmacy to work with them to address the issue. If it is found that an entity acting under the guise of a pharmacy has exceed their state-regulated authority, then the state Boards of Pharmacy should suspend the license of the pharmacy until it complies with state laws and regulations governing compounding or meets FDA standards for manufacturing and registers with the FDA. All parties involved must make certain that the state Boards of Pharmacy are adequately staffed, trained, and funded to effectively regulate compounding.

NCPA encourages state Boards of Pharmacy to require uniform compliance with USP 797 in order to provide more uniform production standards. As such, every state will be assured that resident and non-resident pharmacies alike are all in compliance with these USP standards.

Compounds Are Prepared Based on Prescriptions or on Anticipation of Demand

In most cases, compounded medications must originate from a prescription for a specific patient from a health care professional and are made specifically for an individual patient's needs. In other instances, pharmacists participate in anticipatory compounding where they anticipate a demand that a physician might have for a compounded drug based on historical prescribing patterns. In order to preserve access to these vital compounded medications, pharmacies should not be hindered in their ability to engage in anticipatory compounding as long as it is reasonable and based on a historical pattern of prescriptions received by that pharmacy or for specific patients served by that pharmacy.

Compounding should not be defined by the quantity of medications produced or to where the medications are shipped. Compounding should be defined as the preparation of medications upon receipt of a prescription, or, where in reasonable quantities, in anticipation of need for a medication based upon historical patterns.

To the contrary, compounding should not be defined by nuances such as type of product (i.e. sterile and non-sterile) as risk and complexity of compounding is not solely dependent upon product type; quantity of product made as a pharmacy can produce a significant number of compounded medications and not be a manufacturer as long as the pharmacy is making these medications based on individual prescriptions or in anticipation of need based on historical patterns; or interstate commerce as a pharmacy may legitimately ship to more than one state as long as the pharmacy makes the medications being shipped based on individual prescriptions or in anticipation of need based on historical patterns.

Clear Lines of Communication Between the FDA and State Boards of Pharmacy Are Needed

The FDA should share all inspection data in a timely fashion with state Boards of Pharmacy. Furthermore, FDA should communicate to state Boards of Pharmacy whether the response from the entity inspected addresses all concerns and is sufficient without necessary further action or whether further action is needed to address these concerns. The FDA should strengthen the communication between its regional offices and the states. In addition, FDA should utilize all existing authority and resources in developing and sharing data with states. In order to address the failure in communication in the past, FDA must utilize, and strengthen if necessary, all existing portals and resources in order to produce the needed data sharing to increase communication between the states and FDA.

In Conclusion

While discussing what new regulations should be undertaken to prevent this tragedy in the future, before expanding federal authority it is imperative that Congress look at whether current laws and regulations are being properly enforced. NCPA urges the Committee to preserve the authority of state Boards of Pharmacy over compounding by defining any new category with FDA oversight in a very limited and narrowly targeted manner. In addition, any legislation must not be used to facilitate a broad expansion of FDA power over the historically state-regulated practice of pharmaceutical compounding.

NCPA is committed to working with Members of Congress in order to make certain that a tragedy such as the New England Compounding Center does not occur in the future while also preserving patients' access to customized and safe compounded medications. Thank you for inviting me to testify and to share the viewpoints of independent community pharmacy.

INDEX

D

E

Q

R

S